# Physiology of Speech Production

# Physiology of Speech Production

## An Introduction for Speech Scientists

# W. J. HARDCASTLE

*Department of Linguistics*
*The University of Reading*
*Whiteknights*
*Reading, England*

1976

ACADEMIC PRESS
LONDON · NEW YORK · SAN FRANCISCO
*A Subsidiary of Harcourt Brace Jovanovich Publishers*

ACADEMIC PRESS INC. (LONDON) LTD
24–28 Oval Road,
London NW1

*U.S. Edition published by*
ACADEMIC PRESS INC.
111 Fifth Avenue,
New York, New York 10003

Library of Congress Catalog Card Number: 76–25698
ISBN: 0–12–324950–3

Text set in 11/12 pt. Monotype Baskerville, printed by letterpress,
in Great Britain at The Pitman Press, Bath

# Preface

The last few years have seen a resurgence of interest in the dynamics of articulatory activity during speech production within all those disciplines concerned with speech and language science, such as phonetics, linguistics and speech pathology. One of the research aims in this area, which, because of its potential theoretical importance, has attracted particular attention, is an attempt to specify which features of the speech production process are language-specific, i.e. constrained by the linguistic rules of the particular language, and which features are language universals, i.e. constrained by our anatomical and physiological make-up. Before we can even adequately begin to answer this question we need to know how the speech mechanism functions: how the various articulators move under the influence of muscular contractions, and how movements of the different articulatory organs such as the tongue, lips, mandible, soft palate etc. are co-ordinated by the nervous system of the body.

The aim of the book is basically to provide the speech scientist (especially the phonetician and speech pathologist) with an introductory survey of the functions of the various organs involved in speech production, and the control of these organs by the nervous system. It is hoped that such information will be used as a starting point in the development of an adequately comprehensive theory of linguistic performance. It is hoped also that the material in this book will help towards providing a basic theoretical framework for research in experimental phonetics, particularly when techniques such as electromyography and cinefluorography investigating physiological aspects of speech production are involved.

The book differs from most texts on the physiology of speech production in that it contains primarily only information which is relevant for speech scientists. Detailed discussions of a medical nature are avoided, and certain areas such as the anatomy and physiology of the central nervous system are touched upon only very briefly, in view of the limited scope of the book. However, some aspects of sensori-motor control systems of the body, for example the neuromuscular spindle system, are treated at some length because of their potentially important implications in the serial ordering and motor control of speech production. Although a certain amount of anatomical information concerning the origins, courses and insertions of muscles is offered, the emphasis throughout the book is on the functional activity of the speech organs. For this purpose, use is made of schematic-type diagrams showing probable directions of movements of articulatory organs under the influence of muscular contractions, rather than anatomically accurate pictorial illustrations of muscles. Where it is felt useful to consult the latter type illustrations, the reader is referred to standard works on anatomy from time to time throughout the text. Where relevant, the results of recent experimental phonetic research, particularly electromyographic research on various muscles during speech production, are mentioned.

The book follows a logical sequence. The first two chapters deal with general principles of neurophysiology, particularly the physiology of the peripheral nervous system, and the basic mechanical properties of skeletal muscle fibres as the basis for movement. In these areas I have relied heavily on standard reference works in anatomy and physiology, and a wide range of more specialist research articles often very recently published. The next three chapters deal with, respectively, the physiology of the respiratory system, the larynx and the articulators in the oral cavity. The muscular basis of movements of the various speech organs is discussed in some detail. In this final chapter some suggestions are made as to how the physiological framework presented in the book can be utilized in the development of a physiological theory of phonetics.

I am indebted to a large number of colleagues who offered helpful criticism and advice concerning the material in this book, especially Dr John Laver, University of Edinburgh, Professor Klaus Kohler, Dr W. Barry and Professor E. Witzleb, University of Kiel, and Professor David Crystal and Mr Peter Roach, University of Reading.

I owe special thanks also to my wife Francesca for her patience and consideration during the writing of the book and for helping me with the proof-reading, and to Fr. Else Eldagson for typing the manuscript.

*W. J. Hardcastle*                                                    *August 1976*

# Glossary of Technical Terms Used*

Abduct: To move away from the median position, as in abduction of the vocal cords.

Actin: A protein present within the filaments of striated muscle.

Action-potential: Electrical energy generated in nerve or muscle tissue during excitation.

Adduct: To move towards the median position, as in adduction of the vocal cords.

Afferent nerve: Conducting towards the central nervous system (CNS). The opposite of efferent. Also called sensory nerve.

All-or-none law: Pertaining to the general property of nerves and muscles whose individual fibres react maximally or remain inactive.

Alpha motoneurone: Large diameter motoneurone innervating extra-fusal muscle fibres.

Alpha rhythm: A rhythmic electrical potential recorded from the surface of the brain using the technique of Electroencephalography.

Alveolus: In the lungs, the smallest air space.

Angle: Point where a structure abruptly changes direction, e.g. angle of rib.

Ansa: A loop, e.g. of a nerve.

Antagonist muscle: Muscle which relaxes to enable the protagonist muscles to operate and which is capable, by contraction, of opposing the movement.

Aponeurosis: A tendinous sheet covering a muscle or extending from it to the attachment of the muscle, e.g. abdominal aponeurosis,

*The sources for this glossary include Cunningham (1972), Kaplan (1971), Zemlin (1968), and Eccles (1973).

palatal aponeurosis.

Autonomic nervous system: Part of the peripheral nervous system (PNS) concerned primarily with non-volitional activities of the body. It consists of groups of nerve cells (ganglia) and their processes lying entirely outside the CNS and often arranged in complicated loose meshworks (plexuses) unlike the compact bundles of nerve fibres which constitute the cranial and spinal nerves.

Axon: A nerve fibre.

Basilar membrane: A membrane of the inner ear which supports the Organ of Corti.

Cartilage: A non-vascular white elastic substance, softer and more flexible than bone, often attached to articular bone surfaces, and forming certain parts of the skeleton.

Cervical nerve: *See* Spinal nerve.

Co-articulation: The influence of a phonetic context upon a given speech segment. In a sequence such as ABC if B exerts an influence on C it is called left-to-right or progressive assimilation, if B exerts an influence on A it is called right-to-left or regressive assimilation.

Condyle: A knuckle. A smooth rounded eminence covered with articular cartilage, e.g. condyle of mandible.

Cornu: A horn-shaped structure, e.g. cornu of hyoid bone.

Coronal: A vertical, or cut from side to side, dividing the structure into front and back parts.

Costal: Pertaining to the ribs.

Cranial nerves: Part of the peripheral nervous system, the cranial nerves arise symmetrically in the brain stem and, with the exception of the tenth cranial nerve, are distributed mainly in the head and neck region. The names of the various nerves are as follows: I olfactory, II optic, III oculomotor, IV trochlear, V trigeminal, VI abducent, VII facial, VIII vestibulo-cochlear, IX glossopharyngeal, X vagus, XI accessory, XII hypoglossal.

Cutaneous: Pertaining to the skin.

Decussate: To cross over, as nerves or muscle fibres.

Dorsal: In the coronal plane, the anterior aspect or nearest the front of the body. With reference to the tongue, pertaining to the upper surface (dorsum).

Dorsal root: Referring to sensory afferent nerve fibres which pass through the dorsal (posterior) part of the spinal medulla.

Efferent nerve: Conducting from a central region to the periphery. Also called motor nerve.

Electromyography (EMG): A technique for recording the electrical potentials associated with muscular activity.

End-organ: A terminal structure of a nerve, also called sensory receptor. Types of end-organ are Krause's end-bulbs, "free-endings", Meissner's corpuscles, etc.

End-plate: *See* Motor end-plate.

Epithelium: The covering of the skin and mucous membrane, consisting entirely of cells of various forms and arrangements.

Exteroceptors: Sensory receptors situated on the surface of the body conveying to the CNS information concerning the environment. They include tactile and taste receptors.

Extrafusal: Referring to the normal fibres which make up the contractile bulk of voluntary or skeletal muscle. The term extrafusal is used to distinguish these regular muscle fibres from intrafusal fibres, the thinner specialized fibres present within neuromuscular spindles.

Facial nerve: Cranial nerve VII. A mixed nerve (i.e. one containing both efferent and afferent fibres) which communicates throughout its course with many other nerves. Some of the motor fibres of this nerve supply the posterior belly of the digastricus, the stylohyoideus, and the muscles of the lips.

Fascia: A fibrous connective tissue which encases the body beneath the skin, and separates muscle fibre bundles from each other.

Feedback: A term borrowed from radio technology to mean the diversion of a small part of the output to control the input. It occurs both in natural and man-made systems.

Fibril: A thread-like component of a fibre.

Fixator muscle: Muscle which provides a fixed, stable base from which other muscles can contract.

Flagelliform: Shaped like a whip or lash.

Foramen: An opening or perforation in a bone, e.g. mandibular foramen.

Fossa: A shallow depression.

Fusiform: Spindle-shaped.

Fusimotor: Same as gamma efferent.

Gamma nerve fibres: Also called gamma efferent, or fusimotor fibres. The motor nerve fibres which terminate on the intrafusal muscle fibres of neuromuscular spindles. The gamma fibres are of smaller diameter than the alpha efferent fibres to normal muscle, and may have a lower threshold to excitation within the motor cortex.

Gamma loop system: Mechanism whereby movement is not initiated directly by activation of normal alpha motoneurones but by initial activation of the small gamma fibres which supply the intrafusal muscle fibres of neuromuscular spindles, and reflexly cause firing in the alpha neurones. The operative path is gamma motoneurones → muscle spindles → Ia fibres → alpha motoneurones → extrafusal muscle contraction.

Ganglion: A collection of nerve cell bodies lying outside the brain or spinal medulla. The dorsal root ganglion contains the cell bodies of afferent neurones.

Glossopharyngeal nerve: Cranial nerve IX. It is a mixed nerve which emerges in the brain stem from the groove posterior to the olive. Some of the sensory fibres supply the mucous membrane of the pharynx and the back part of the tongue. A motor branch innervates the stylopharyngeus muscle.

Gyrus: A hill or convolution of the cerebral cortex, as opposed to sulcus or depression.

Hamulus: Any hook-shaped process. The pterygoid hamulus is a paired process of the pterygoid bone of the skull.

Histology (adj. histological): The branch of anatomy concerned with the minute structure of the tissues.

Humerus: The bone of the arm.

Hypoglossal nerve: Cranial nerve XII. Mainly a motor nerve which innervates the intrinsic and extrinsic muscles of the tongue.

Iliohyogastric nerve: Highest branch of the first lumbar nerve (see Spinal nerves) some of the fibres of which innervate the muscles of the abdominal wall.

Ilio-inguinal nerve: One of the two branches given off from the first lumbar nerve (the other being the iliohyogastric nerve) the motor fibres of which supply some of the muscles of the abdominal wall.

Inguinal: Pertaining to the groin.

Innervation: The supplying of any organ with nerve fibres.

Innervation ratio: Referring to the number of muscle fibres innervated by branches of the single motoneurone within a motor unit. In general, large, slow-moving muscles have high innervation ratios (i.e. a large number of muscle fibres per motor unit) and small, fast muscles such as the tongue and eye muscles have low innervation ratios (i.e. small number of muscle fibres per motor unit).

Insertion: The area of attachment of a muscle to the structure it moves.

Interdigitate: The interlocking of similar parts, as muscle fibres from different muscles.

Intrafusal: Referring to the thin, specialized muscle fibres present within a neuromuscular spindle and arranged in parallel with the regular or extrafusal fibres of the muscle.

Ion: An atom or group of atoms, which, due to outside force, has lost or gained one or more orbital electrons and thus becomes capable of conducting electricity.

Keratin: A protein which can be deposited on a tissue to make it rough and horny.

Kinesthetic: A general term referring to the sense of movement and/ or position of parts of the body. Kinesthetic sensation probably results from an integration in the CNS of information supplied by tactile and proprioceptive receptors.

Lamina: A plate or sheet. Hence lamina propria: sheets of tissue.

Lateral inhibition: A funneling action of the responses of some receptor organs whereby smaller stimulus effects are inhibited and stronger effects are collected into a common pathway to enable a stimulus to be precisely located.

Ligament: A band of flexible, elastic, dense fibrous tissue, connecting the articular ends of the bones or cartilages. Sometimes found in a capsule, completely enveloping the joint.

Lumbar nerve: *See* Spinal nerve.

Maxilla: The upper jaw.

Mechanoreceptors: Receptors responding to pressure, stretch and mechanical forces.

Micron: (Sign $\mu$). One millionth of a m i.e. one thousandth of a mm.

Monosynaptic reflex: A reflex arc which comprises only one afferent and one efferent neurone with no interneurones, therefore has only one synapse.

Motor end-plate: The specialized part of a muscle fibre forming the junction between the muscle fibre and motor nerve.

Motor unit: The unit subserving muscular movement, consisting of one motoneurone and the muscle fibres innervated by branches of that neurone.

Mucous membrane: Epithelium upon a basement membrane with a subcutaneus tissue. It lines the inside of the oral cavity, and secretes a viscid watery substance called mucus.

Muscle spindle: Specialized encapsulated bundle of fine muscle fibres (intrafusal fibres) responding to changes in length of the main muscle.

Myelinated nerve fibre: Nerve fibres surrounded by fatty sheaths. Also called medullated nerve fibres.

Myodynamic: Pertaining to the contractions and movements of muscles.

Myofibrils: The long, thin elements about a micron in diameter which make up the contractile structure of a muscle fibre.

Myosin: A protein present within the filaments of striated muscle. An energy-liberating chemical reaction between myosin and adenosine triphosphate (ATP) and is supposed to be associated with muscular contraction.

Organ of Corti: The end-organ of hearing, situated on the basilar membrane in the inner ear and containing the hair cells that respond to sound waves.

Origin: The place of attachment of a muscle that remains relatively fixed during contraction.

Papilla: A small, nipple-like eminence. Plural: papillae, e.g. papillae of the tongue.

Pectoral: Pertaining to the chest and shoulder: pectoral girdle = shoulder girdle, pectoral muscles (here) = shoulder muscles.

Pennate: Feather-like.

Periodontal membrane: Special membrane surrounding the root of a tooth.

Petrous: Hard, dense bone, e.g. petrous portion of the temporal bone of the skull.

Plexus: A network of nerves or veins.

Polysynaptic: Referring to a neural pathway containing a number of synaptic connections in series.

Primary ending: Also called an annulospiral ending because of its histological shape. A receptor organ attached to the central part of intrafusal fibres registering stretch on the neuromuscular spindle. Neural discharge in the primary ending is transmitted to the CNS via large diameter Group Ia afferent fibres.

Process: A prominence of a bone or cartilage, e.g. transverse process of vertebrae.

Proprioceptive: Pertaining to sensory information supplied to the CNS from the muscles spindles, joint receptors, and Golgi tendon organs.

Protagonist: Also called prime mover. Referring to muscle(s) that effect the actual movement that occurs.

Ramus: Branch of a vessel or nerve, also section of a bone, e.g. ramus of mandible.

Raphe: A line of union between the members of a bilaterally symmetrical structure.

Refractory period, absolute: The period of time (usually about 0·8 msec) following a nerve impulse during which it is impossible to generate a second impulse.

Refractory period, relative: The time following the absolute refractory period during which a stronger stimulus is required to initiate a nerve impulse, the nerve impulse being smaller and slower (Eccles, 1973).

Renshaw cells: Nuclei located in the medial part of the ventral horns of the spinal medulla, which send axons to neighbouring moto-neurones and inhibit their activity.

Sagittal: Pertaining to the antero-posterior median plane of the body.

Secondary ending: Also called "flower-spray" ending. Receptor organ located adjacent to the central part of the intrafusal fibres in muscle spindles, responding to stretch on the spindle.

Septum: A partition, e.g. a fibrous septum separating two groups of muscle fibres.

Servo-system: An automatic mechanism in which the output is partly controlled by feeding back a part of the output to the controlling elements.

Skeletal muscle: Muscle which executes movements initiated by the will, also known as voluntary or striated muscle.

Spatial summation: Summation of synaptic actions arising from convergence on a neurone of pathways coming from different sites (Eccles, 1973).

Sphincter: A muscle arranged around an opening to constrict or dilate the passageway.

Spinal medulla: The spinal cord, situated within the vertebral column and giving rise to the spinal nerves.

Spinal nerve: The spinal nerves are attached to the spinal medulla and pass out between the vertebrae. They comprise usually 31 pairs grouped as cervical (written as C1–C8), thoracic (T1–T12), lumbar (L1–L5), sacral (S1–S5), and coccygeal (Co) according to the vertebrae between which they emerge.

Stretch reflex: The feedback of information from muscle receptors (e.g. spindles) concerning the tensions of these muscles and the adaptive changes in the tone of the same muscles.

Striated muscle: Voluntary muscle so-called because it shows under a microscope characteristic transverse striations alternatively pale and dark.

Styloid process: A downward projecting spur from the temporal bone of the skull serving as the origin of many muscles (e.g. stylohyoideus, styloglossus, etc.) and ligaments.

Sulcus: A depression of the cerebral cortex, as opposed to gyrus, or hill.

Symphysis: The point of union between bones that were originally separate, e.g. mandibular symphysis.

Synapse: The region where two neurones meet and where impulses are passed from one to the other.

Synergistic muscle: Muscle which assists other muscles (either protagonist or antagonist) in effecting a particular movement.

Temporomandibular joint: A complex joint connecting the lower jaw to the temporal bone of the skull.

Tendon: A connective tissue band which connects a muscle with a bone.

Tetanus: A fusion of discrete individual muscular contractions.

Thoracic nerve: *See* Spinal nerves.

Trigeminal nerve: The fifth (V) cranial nerve, which has both sensory and motor fibres. The main branches are the ophthalmic, maxillary, and mandibular branches. The mandibular branch is concerned with general sensation in the anterior part of the mouth and innervation of the mandibular muscles.

Vagus: Cranial nerve X. The vagus is a mixed nerve so-called because of its wandering course throughout the head, neck, and abdominal regions. A superior laryngeal branch supplies the motor innervation of the cricothyroideus muscle and part of the constrictor pharyngis inferior. The intrinsic laryngeal muscles are supplied by a loop called the recurrent nerve which arises from the vagus below the larynx. A pharyngeal branch passes into the pharyngeal plexus from which the muscles of the pharynx and soft palate (except the stylopharyngeus and tensor veli palatini) are supplied.

Ventral: In the coronal plane, the posterior aspect, or nearest the back of the body. With reference to the tongue, away from the dorsum. Opposite of dorsal.

Ventral root: Referring to the motor efferent nerve fibres which pass through the ventral (anterior) part of the spinal medulla.

Zygomatic arch: The prominent bone on the side of the face, or cheek, produced by the zygomatic process of the temporal bone fusing anteriorly with the zygoma or malar bone.

# Contents

## 1
## General Neurophysiology of Speech Production

## 2
## Biomechanical Constraints on Muscular Activity

## 3
## The Physiology of Respiratory Activity

## 4
## The Physiology of the Larynx

## 5
## The Physiology of Articulatory Organs in the Vocal Tract

## 6
## Concluding Remarks: Approaches to a Physiological Theory of Phonetics

# 1
# General Neurophysiology of Speech Production

## I.  The Nervous System of the Body

For most descriptive purposes, the nervous system of the body is divided into central and peripheral parts, the central part or central nervous system (CNS) comprising the brain and spinal medulla and the peripheral part or peripheral nervous system (PNS), the nerves. However, as Cunningham (1972, p. 581) points out, the division is somewhat arbitrary because both parts are essential components of a single functioning unit and cannot be clearly separated from each other on anatomical grounds.

A detailed description of the anatomy of the CNS is clearly beyond the scope of this introductory book, although it may be useful at this stage to briefly outline some of the more important anatomical landmarks in the brain, which will be referred to from time to time throughout the text (for more detailed accounts see Cunningham, 1972; Sutton, 1971; Chusid and McDonald, 1967; Ranson and Clark, 1964).

A brief description of the CNS can begin with the spinal medulla, situated within the vertebral column, and the brain stem, which is anatomically really an extension of the spinal medulla, consisting principally of a number of relatively well-defined structures such as the medulla oblongata, pons, midbrain (or mesencephalon), and thalamus. The nuclei of the cranial nerves which are important for the production of speech, are situated at various points throughout the brain stem (Sutton, 1971, pp. 47–59).

Just posterior to the medulla oblongata at the head of the spinal column is an important structure, the cerebellum or "little brain". It has been described as a neuronal machine (Eccles *et al.*, 1967), which processes information received from both the periphery of the body and from the motor centres of the cortex to enable precise co-ordination of muscular movements to take place.

Above the brain stem are the two cerebral hemispheres, which together make up more than 80% of the total brain weight. It is here that the most complex bodily activities such as speech production are

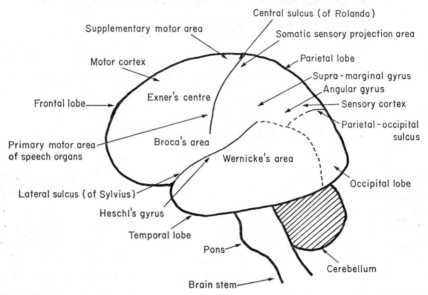

Fig. 1 The lateral surface of the left cerebral hemisphere in a right-handed person showing some of the main structural parts and the positions of the various "speech centres".

initiated. Each hemisphere can be divided into four main lobes, the frontal, parietal, occipital and temporal lobes on the basis of three well-defined creases or sulci; the central sulcus (of Rolando), the lateral sulcus (of Sylvius), and the parieto-occipital sulcus. Figure 1 shows a schematic diagram of the left cerebral hemisphere (which is generally regarded as being the dominant hemisphere for speech production in a right-handed person) illustrating the spatial relationship of the major landmarks. The central sulcus has great functional significance in that it divides the cortical areas of the brain into an anterior part, which is mainly efferent or motor in function, and a posterior part, which has afferent or sensory functions.

Various specific areas of the dominant cerebral cortex are generally regarded to be of prime importance for speech and language (Whitaker, 1969, pp. 30–32). These are the so-called speech centres, damage to any of which frequently causes certain fairly well-defined disruptions in speech. The areas of importance include Broca's area, Exner's centre, Heschl's gyrus, Angular gyrus, Supra-marginal gyrus, Wernicke's area, and the Supplementary motor area (see Fig. 1). These areas have been determined largely by electrical stimulation and by operative excision (e.g. Penfield and Roberts, 1959; Luria, 1966).

Although considerably complex, the general anatomy of the CNS is relatively uncontroversial, with most investigations agreeing at least on the placement of the main neural structures. Almost nothing, however, is known about the integrative functions of the various neural structures, particularly during complex bodily activities such as speech production. The main reason for our lack of knowledge in this area is quite clearly the relative inaccessibility of the normal live human brain to direct investigations, forcing us to rely heavily on inferences from experiments involving animals, or by studying speech and language in patients with various types of brain damage. We can, however, at least in theory, throw considerable light on the physiological complexities of the CNS by studying closely different aspects of the more peripheral neural mechanisms, which are relatively more accessible to experimental investigation. Most attention in this book will therefore be focused on the peripheral nervous system with occasional reference to hypothetical central mechanisms where relevant.

The PNS is broadly divisible on an anatomical basis into three parts:

(i) the twelve cranial nerves (referred to as I–XII), which arise from the brain stem and pass through the skull to be distributed predominantly in the head and neck region;
(ii) the spinal nerves, which are attached to the spinal medulla and innervate the trunk and limbs;
(iii) the autonomic nervous system, which consists of nerve cells and their processes lying outside the CNS and is concerned with non-volitional activities such as supplying the blood vessels, sweat glands, viscera, heart, etc.

It is the cranial nerves which are most relevant for a discussion of speech physiology, and therefore will be the main subject of the following discussion.

The cranial nerve system innervates most of the muscles involved in speech articulation; it consists mostly of "mixed" nerves, that is, those containing a large number of both efferent and afferent nerve fibres, the former sending neural commands in the form of trains of impulses out from the CNS to muscle fibres, and the latter transmitting back to the CNS information derived from the receptor organs in the skin, mucosa and muscles. It is thus essential in understanding the myodynamic control of speech to distinguish between the efferent (motor) system and the afferent (sensory) system.

## II. The Efferent (Motor) System

### A. Structure of the Motoneurone

In order to understand how muscles are innervated, it is necessary to describe first the structure of an efferent- or moto- neurone. Figure 2 shows a schematic diagram of a typical motoneurone. The important functional parts are the cell body, nucleus, the dendrites attached to the body, and the long process of the axon with its various branches or collaterals. The collaterals and axons terminate either on other neurones or on muscle fibres at regions known as end-plates. The axon is usually referred to as the nerve fibre and can vary greatly in length, from fractions of a millimetre to several centimetres long. Dendrites are nerve processes similar to the axon but they conduct the neural impulse towards the nucleus, whereas the axons normally conduct the neural impulse away from the nucleus.

On the surface of the cell body and dendrites of each neurone there are a number of specialized junctions or synapses where connections are made with other neurones. The nervous system can thus be regarded as a complex interconnecting network of neurones, each one connected to many, sometimes thousands, of other nerve cells, all capable of conducting neural impulses.

### B. Propagation of the Neural Impulse

The key to an understanding of how neural impulses, in the form of electrical potentials, are transmitted along the nerve fibre, lies in the properties of a semi-permeable membrane which surrounds the axon process. It appears that this membrane is selectively permeable, i.e.

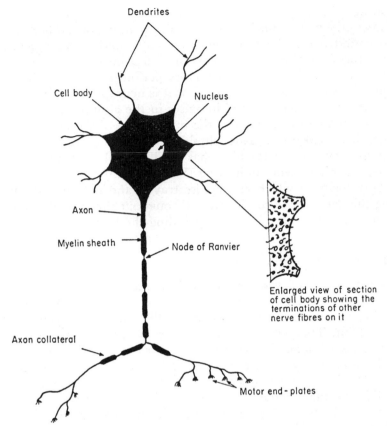

Fig. 2 A typical motoneurone showing some of the main functional parts (after Cunningham, 1972, p. 587).

it allows some chemical substances to pass more readily than others. In an unstimulated resting condition, positive potassium ions are allowed to pass out through the membrane, and this results in the inside of the axon being negatively charged with respect to the outside. During excitation, the membrane momentarily becomes much more permeable to sodium ions resulting in an ion-exchange process that reverses the negative membrane potential. Current will then flow immediately to the next negative region of the membrane so triggering the generation of another action-potential. The neural impulses in the form of action potential "spikes" thus travel down the axon as a series of pulses (Hodgkin, 1964). During excitation, the size of the stimulus is not reflected in the size of the action-potential but in the frequency of the spikes transmitted along the axon. The greater the stimulus the higher the frequency of spikes.

During the passage of the action-potential (lasting usually about 0·8 msec) the membrane is incapable of responding to another stimulus. This period is called the absolute refractory period. Stimuli arriving within this critical period will have no effect on the depolarization of the membrane. The absolute refractory period principle has important implications for theories of hearing, as it is neurophysiologically impossible for synchronous firing of impulses in the auditory nerve fibres to occur at frequencies as high as the upper limit of the normal hearing range, i.e. 20,000 Hz. This physiological limitation on maximum firing frequencies in nerve fibres has resulted in the generally accepted place-and-volley theory of hearing (Wever, 1949).

The velocity at which an impulse travels and its transmission time along the axon varies considerably throughout the cranial nerves and depends on a number of factors, including the following points.

## 1. The Diameter of the Axon

It is generally believed that there is a direct relationship between conduction velocity and axon diameter; larger axons conducting impulses at a higher velocity (Hursh, 1939; Boyd and Davey, 1966; Katz, 1966). The peripheral nerve fibres are usually classified on the basis of their conduction velocities into groups labelled A, B and C, the A group being further subdivided into alpha, beta, gamma and delta. The classification scheme was proposed by Erlanger and Gasser (1937). The main motor fibres to muscles are largest and have the highest conduction velocity; they come in the alpha category of group A. Some of these large axons send impulses that travel as fast as 100 metres a second.

There also seems to be some relationship between conduction velocity of neurones and their threshold to electrical excitation. Large, high-velocity cells seem to have a lower threshold to electrical stimulation (Erlanger and Gasser, 1937; Roberts, 1966, p. 76) and so may be recruited more readily by input from the motor cortex than smaller low-velocity cells.

## 2. The Type of Membrane

Thicker diameter axons can have a special sheath consisting largely of cells called Schwann cells wrapped closely about the membrane forming part of a layer of fatty material known as myelin. The myelin coating is not continuous but has gaps in it called nodes of Ranvier (see Fig. 2).

Ion exchange during excitation of the neurone takes place only at these points: thus the action-potential leaps, as it were, from node to node. This enables the impulse to travel along the fibre quicker than would be possible if it were unmyelinated. The axons of cranial nerves innervating the speech musculature are usually myelinated for most of their length so are capable of fast activation.

## 3. The Length of the Axon

Obviously, the transmission time of the impulse depends on the length of the nerve fibres. All other things being equal, the longer the axon the longer the time taken for the neural impulse to reach its destination. Lenneberg (1967) illustrates schematically the difference in length of peripheral nerves innervating the speech musculature. He hypothesizes that, because of these different lengths, the firing order in the motor nuclei of these nerves may at times be different from the order of events occurring at the periphery. An index of the propagation time of neural impulses along the axon may be obtained by dividing the length of the fibre by its diameter. The order of latency for the cranial nerves innervating the speech musculature would then be in the following progression (those with shortest latency first): facial nerve (supplying the muscles of the lips), trigeminal nerve (supplying the pterygoideus and mylohyoideus muscles of the jaw), accessory nerve (supplying the muscles of the pharynx), hypoglossal nerve (supplying the muscles of the tongue), recurrent laryngeal branch of vagus (supplying the intrinsic muscles of the larynx). The latencies may have important consequences for the temporal ordering of different articulatory organs during speech.

## 4. Temperature of the Axon

Another factor having an effect on the conduction velocity is the temperature of the nerve fibre; the higher the temperature, the more rapidly a given impulse is propagated along the length of the axon. This factor is probably not so important for humans, as our body temperature remains fairly constant.

## C. Synaptic Connections between Neurones

When a motor command in the form of trains of impulses is initiated in the CNS, the impulses never travel via one nerve cell only, but traverse many synaptic junctions before reaching the periphery. In this way the original signal to the muscles is constantly modified due to the influence of neighbouring cells. At each synaptic junction, a chemical substance called acetylcholine is released, facilitating the transmission of the electrical potentials. The transmission process does not occur instantaneously, however, there is a delay called a synaptic delay of about 0·4 msec, so, in general, the more synapses there are in a motor command pathway the longer will be the time for the impulses to reach the muscles.

When a single impulse arrives at a synaptic junction it produces a small transient electrical effect of about 1 mvolt which lasts for 10 to 20 msec. This small electrical charge is not enough to effect the synaptic transmission by setting up an impulse spike potential in the post-synaptic neurone. It requires the concerted effort of a number of neurones to produce the necessary voltage (about 10 mvolt) to discharge the impulse across the synapse. This concerted effort is known as the principle of summation (Eccles, 1958).

Many of the neurones making synapses are excitatory, that is, they facilitate the passing of the trans-synaptic electrical charges. Some, however, are inhibitory generating reverse electrical charges (e.g. more negative instead of more positive membrane potential) and so resisting transmission of the impulse. For example, during articulation of a high back vowel such as [u], motor commands are probably sent to the tongue elevator muscles such as the styloglossus, while at the same time the motoneurones supplying the antagonist muscles which depress the tongue such as the hyoglossus are relatively inhibited. Thus, in general, under the influence of a number of incoming impulses, a neurone must sum the opposing synaptic effects and can fire only when its net excitation exceeds the critical level.

The process of spatial summation contributes greatly to the versatility of the nervous system. If excitation at each synapse were obligatory, movement would become stereotyped and incapable of modification. As it is, because of the ability of the CNS to regulate the firing of excitatory and inhibitory cells, usually by means of special interneurones, movements can be continually modulated and varied according to prevailing conditions. The process of spatial summation also provides an explanation of why certain responses will usually be made only if two or more circumstances coexist. Thus in closing off the nasal from the oral passageway, the superior pharyngeal constrictor muscle may perhaps contract only in unison with the tensor and levator muscles (Van Riper and Irwin, 1958, p. 383).

Once an impulse has succeeded in passing through a synapse the threshold to future excitation at that synapse is lowered. This means it is then easier for future impulses to pass through the synapse; they are facilitated. The detailed biochemical processes whereby this facilitation is made possible is still not certain but most researchers agree that a permanent chemical change takes place in the region of the synapse (probably involving the release of an increased amount of acetylcholine) as soon as an impulse passes. Because of this facilitation process it is possible to set up neural pathways in the CNS where some courses are favoured over others and in time become stereotyped. Much of speech consists of stereotyped, almost automatic utterances which can be "primed" and "triggered off as a whole" (Craik, 1947, p. 56; Lashley, 1951, p. 188).

## D. Innervation of Skeletal Muscle by the Motor System

### 1. Structure of Voluntary Muscle

Every movement of the articulatory organs depends on contraction of muscle, which in turn is mediated by the motoneurones. Voluntary, or striated, muscle is made up of individual muscle fibres of varying sizes and shapes; cylindrically shaped fibres are usually short, while flagelliform fibres are longer and usually extend the whole length of the muscle. The diameter of the individual fibres varies from about 10 to 100 microns (1 micron = 0·001 mm), and their length can be anything up to several centimetres (Huxley, 1965).

Within most striated muscles, there are groups of smaller fibres running parallel with the main muscle fibres but gathered together in special receptor organs, called muscle spindles. These smaller fibres are usually separately innervated from the main fibres and are called intrafusal fibres to distinguish them from the main, or extrafusal fibres. The innervation of intrafusal fibres is of some functional importance in the control of speech production and will be discussed more fully later.

The individual muscle fibres and so in turn the whole muscle can respond in a number of ways when an appropriate stimulus is applied to it; it may shorten if it can; it may develop tension against a resistance; or it may show an increased resistance to extension. The stimulus comes from the nerve fibre supplying the muscle fibre at a region called the muscle end-plate or neuro-muscular junction. Most of the motoneurones supplying extrafusal fibres are large myelinated fibres classified as type alpha while smaller gamma fibres have also been found in the motor nerves (Leksell, 1945). It is usually thought that these gamma fibres are responsible for innervating the intrafusal fibres but there is a possibility that intrafusal fibres are supplied by large or alpha type fibres as well (Matthews, 1964, p. 257).

The stimuli which pass through the alpha and gamma motor fibres have their origin, broadly speaking, in a region of the cerebral cortex anterior to the central sulcus. This region is generally referred to as the "motor" cortex. It is interesting to note that different parts of the body are topographically represented in specific regions of this area; motor areas subserving the body from the toes to the head occur along a line running from the top of the central sulcus down to the lateral sulcus. Those areas of the body requiring considerable delicacy of control, for example the tongue and larynx, occupy relatively large parts of the motor cortex area.

The motoneurones subserving voluntary movement are generally regarded as being the large pyramidal cells of Betz which are situated in one of the layers of the motor cortex. Impulses from these cells are continually modified by synaptic connections from cells in other areas of the brain before they are projected upon sub-cortical areas and finally to the muscles themselves. It is not known how a voluntary movement is initiated although it is fairly well established now that a large number of cortical and sub-cortical structures in different parts of the brain participate actively in the creation of the movement.

## 2. The Neuro-muscular Junction and Muscle Action-potentials

When the propagated action-potential from the motor fibre impinges on the region of the neuro-muscular junction, a complex sequence of electrochemical processes takes place resulting in an electrical muscle action-potential spreading along the muscle fibre causing it to contract or "twitch" just once. A detailed account of the transmission of nerve impulses at the neuro-muscular junction can be found in Eccles (1973), and in Katz (1962). The mechanical twitch does not, however, occur immediately the action-potential arrives at the junction; there is usually a delay of about 2 msec before the twitch occurs, depending on the intrinsic speed of the muscle fibre itself. The propagation of action-potentials constitute the basic electrical phenomena from which electromyographic records are derived.

Usually, the entire fibre does not undergo maximal shortening when activated by a single stimulus. The main reasons for this are the mechanical properties of muscle, including the elastic elements consisting of connective tissues and tendons, etc. For full shortening to occur, the active state of the muscles must be maintained by repetitive stimulation.

Under normal conditions this is what happens; the result is sustained rather than twitch-like muscular activity. This sustained contraction is called tetanic contraction, and it produces shortening of the fibre which may be two or three times as great as the single twitch; thus it is far more efficient.

After contraction of the muscle fibre, there is a short period of time (the refractory period) while the original chemical balance is restored. The frequency of discharge of the action-potential is limited by this refractory period. Impulses arriving too fast (i.e. before the chemical balance is restored) will usually have no effect. In actual muscular contraction, however, this is perhaps avoided by some sort of inhibitory mechanism, for instance, the Renshaw loop control connected to the motoneurones (Roberts, 1966, p. 95).

## 3. The Motor Unit

There are probably more than forty muscles involved in some aspects of the articulatory process, containing several million fibres, and only a fraction of that number myelinated nerve fibres, so obviously each individual muscle fibre cannot each be supplied by a separate nerve fibre. The concept of a motor unit as the functional unit of muscular activity has thus been introduced into physiology (Liddell and Sherrington, 1925; Buller, 1969) the unit consisting of a single motoneurone, its axon, and the group of muscle fibres innervated by branches of this axon. By virtue of the anatomical relationship, electrical activity in the nerve cell of a motor unit leads to activation of all the muscle fibres in that unit. Thus a single impulse arriving via the nerve fibre of a motor unit and impinging on the muscle end-plates of each muscle fibre in that unit will cause all the muscle fibres to contract just once. Increased tension in the muscle will be accompanied by increasing rate of firing of the motor units and a state of tetanic contraction may result.

The number of muscle fibres in a motor unit (the innervation ratio) varies from muscle to muscle according to the role they play in motor activity. In general, muscles requiring delicate adjustments of movement, for example the intrinsic tongue muscles, probably have a low innervation ratio, i.e. a small number of muscle fibres for each motor unit (probably about seven), whereas larger muscles requiring only gross control, e.g. the lower limb muscles, have large innervation ratios (up to 1,700). This, added to the fact that each motor unit is under separate neural control via the controlling motor nerve fibre, means it is possible to achieve delicately controlled tongue configurations, for example in the production of the grooved fricative [s].

Not only does the number of muscle fibres in a motor unit vary, but often also the distribution of motor units throughout the muscle varies. The motor units may be distributed evenly throughout the muscle, but they are often gathered into groups in certain parts of the muscle. This differential distribution is obviously of considerable importance in interpreting the electrical activity at a specific point in the muscle (e.g. by electromyographic techniques).

Since the stimulated muscle fibres in a motor unit either contract or do not — the all-or-none principle — so obviously the motor units supplying a muscle do not normally all work together at the same time. If this were the case, the muscle would contract as a series of violent jerks and controlled precise gradation of contraction as is necessary for certain speech articulations would be impossible. In the course of normal muscular activity, however, the responses of the different motor units are out of phase. This may be due to different thresholds to excitation in the collection of motoneurones for any one particular muscle, the motoneurone pool, or different diameters of nerve fibres carrying impulses to the muscle fibres (Bessou *et al.*, 1963; Henneman *et al.*, 1965). Henneman *et al.* hypothesize an order of recruitment of motor units during a muscular contraction which is dependent upon the size of the motoneurones. Thus in any motoneurone pool there are numbers of motoneurones of different sizes; the sizes being proportional to their threshold to excitation (larger motoneurones being less excitable than smaller ones). According to Henneman, as the force in a muscle increases, motor units of steadily increasing size are recruited, thus resulting in a graded contraction, which is essential, for example in controlling accurate articulatory movements.

To sum up therefore, increase in muscular effort is accompanied by two effects:

    (i)  increase in the repetition frequency of activity cycles in individual motor units, and

   (ii)  increase in the number of units showing activity.

Because of (ii) it turns out that the detailed analysis of electromyographic records from surface electrodes is often highly unreliable because they are composed of so many components virtually indistinguishable from each other. This is particularly true of complex muscular systems such as the tongue, and most electromyographic studies on the tongue using surface electrodes have been severely limited by this fact (MacNeilage and Sholes, 1964).

## III. The Afferent (Sensory) System

### A. General Structure of Sensory Neurones and Receptor Organs

Afferent neurones are similar in general structure to motoneurones but unlike motoneurones, they usually have their nuclei close to the periphery of the body and conduct neural impulses from receptor organs in the skin, mucosa, or muscles, towards the CNS. These receptor organs may be separate receptor cells connected to the sensory fibre or may be dendrite-like terminals of the sensory fibre itself. They act like "biological transducers" (Loewenstein, 1960) generating patterns of neural impulses, which are transmitted back to the CNS, and result in sensations such as heat, cold, touch, pressure, etc. Often each sensory receptor sends messages in only one sensory nerve fibre but single fibres may be connected to a number of receptors in which case the whole group is called a sensory unit. The analogy with the motor unit is quite clear.

Electrophysiological experiments have shown that stimulation of receptors results in a flow of electrical current that excited the nerve fibres. The intensity and duration of the applied stimulus is reflected in the repetition frequency of the electrical potential in the sensory fibre. Thus the message sent to the CNS is coded in terms of a series of identical action-potentials of varying frequency in particular nerve fibres.

A second way in which the intensity of the stimulus affects the afferent discharge is in the number of sensory receptors active. As the stimulus increases, more sensory units become active, a process known as "recruitment of end-organs". A similar process takes place in moto-neurone pools as more and more motor units are recruited during an increase in muscular tension.

### B. Sensory Resources Associated with Speech Production

Sensory receptors associated with speech production are situated in the oral region and in the respiratory system. They can be divided into two general categories according to whether they are normally excited by mechanical or by chemical means. Mechanoreceptors respond to various kinds of mechanical distortion arising, for instance, from the tongue touching the palate or teeth, by generating a depolarizing current in the

sensory fibre (Gray, 1959). Chemoreceptors, such as those responsible
for detecting taste, as their name implies, respond to chemical changes
and as such are probably not important in controlling speech articulation. It should be noted here that there appears to be no direct correlation between specific receptors and sensory modalities such as touch,
pressure, heat, cold, etc. It seems rather that the nature of oral sensation
is determined by the pattern and intensity of nerve impulses and not by
the stimulation of specific receptors (Weddell, 1960; Woodford, 1964).

Most of the oral mucosa and particularly the tongue surface is
supplied with many different types of mechanoreceptors (Grossman
and Hattis, 1967). Although it is probably true to say no two receptors
are identical in size and shape (Ormea and Re, 1959), nevertheless, on
the basis of their morphological structure, a broad classification of
receptors into diffuse ("free") endings and compact ("organized")
endings is sometimes made (Weddell, 1960; Winkelmann, 1960). It has
been tentatively suggested (Hardcastle, 1970) that there may be some
functional significance in this classification for the sensory control of
speech articulation, the free endings, particularly the superficial free
endings, subserving a general sensation of touch, and the organized
endings allowing more discriminative touch—a high degree of tactile
acuity. A clue to the function of the receptor organs may lie in their
morphological structure and their position in the oral mucosa.

The free endings are fine, diffuse overlapping terminal filaments,
which interweave with one another throughout the oral mucosa. They
arise from branching myelinated nerve fibres of varying diameters
which become unmyelinated and form dense networks or plexuses
(Kantner, 1957). Fibres from the superficial plexuses perhaps penetrate
into the epithelium some reaching the most superficial epithelial layers.
It should be noted that there are considerable technical difficulties in
demonstrating the presence of fine nerve fibres in the epithelium; there
is quite a lot of evidence, however, that some fibres do in fact penetrate
at least into the base of the epithelial membrane.

Figure 3 shows a schematic diagram of three nerve fibres showing
overlapping fields of free endings in the oral mucosa. Because of the
network arrangement of fibres, stimulation at any point, for example
point X, will necessarily activate a number of fibres. No two points,
however, come equally within the territory of the same nerve fibres
(see Fig. 3). Thus if the epithelium is touched at X it is within the
receptive area of all three nerve fibres. The pattern of discharge for
area X is therefore unique in that no other point in the whole body is
exactly in that position in the fields of these nerve fibres. Békésy (1967,
p. 38) discusses a principle called lateral inhibition, which enables the

point of stimulation to be localized in the sensory cortex. It is interesting to note that the inhibition is stronger for stimuli with rapid onsets and this produces a greater degree of tactile acuity (Békésy, 1967, p. 46).

The organized sensory receptors, unlike the free endings, are usually well defined morphologically distinct structures, consisting normally of fibrous tissue capsules, through which a nerve fibre pursues a complex

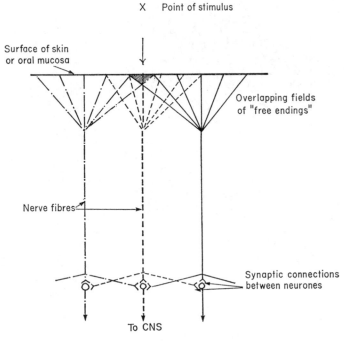

Fig. 3 Three afferent nerve fibres showing overlapping fields of "free endings" at the periphery of the body.

course sometimes dividing into minute fibrils. The structures of two types of encapsulated endings, Krause end-bulbs and Meissner corpuscles, are illustrated diagrammatically in Fig. 4. In general, because of their relatively large size, these organized receptors in the tongue are situated below the superficial free endings particularly in the papillary lamina propria and the subpapillary lamina propria (see Fig. 4). Most of these receptors particularly those of the Meissner corpuscle type respond to the slightest degree of deformation and stop discharging directly the movement ceases. The impulses are discharged through large sensory nerve fibres, measuring on an average 8–10 $\mu$m in diameter. The fibres supplying these receptors are probably of slightly less calibre than alpha motor fibres supplying the main muscle fibres. It may be that these organized receptors responding accurately to different degrees of pressure, may play some important part in sensori-motor co-ordination of speech.

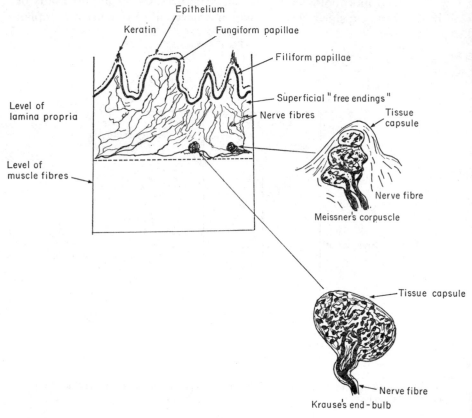

Fig. 4 A highly magnified coronal section through the front part of the tongue, and two types of "organized endings" found frequently in the deeper layers of the lamina propria. (The drawings of the Meissner's corpuscle and Krause's end-bulb are based on sketches in Cunningham 1972.)

The mechanoreceptors so far mentioned are situated in the mucosa throughout the oral region. There are a number of types of receptors, however, which are situated within the oral musculature, in the capsules of joints and present within the periodontal membranes of teeth. The receptors in the muscles and joints respond to stretch on the muscles or movement of the joints, and are usually referred to respectively as muscle spindles and joint receptors. The receptors attached to the periodontal membrane are known as the periodontal receptors. The neurophysiology of joint receptors in the temporomandibular joint, which is the main joint associated with speech articulation in the oral region, has been discussed in detail (Kawamura *et al.*, 1967; Klineberg *et al.*, 1970) so will not be described at length here. Suffice it to say that the joint receptors respond directly to stretching on the capsule in the joints usually caused by the action of the mandibular muscles. Periodontal receptors and muscle spindles probably play an important role in the myodynamic control of speech so they will be discussed at some length.

Periodontal receptors are the fine filament endings situated in the periodontal membrane of teeth and respond to an extremely slight touch on the teeth (Scott and Symons, 1974). As the pressure sense of these receptors is extremely delicate, corresponding in sensitivity to some of the encapsulated receptors in the tongue (Pfaffmann, 1939), they would certainly respond to pressure exerted by the tongue during normal speech articulation, and thus may perhaps play some part in myodynamic control. As far as this writer is aware, the presence and possible importance of periodontal receptors has not been mentioned before in the phonetic literature.

The other type of receptor mentioned, the muscle spindle, has been located in all the muscles involved in speech production, including the laryngeal muscles (Hosokawa, 1961; Sawashima, 1974). Although traditionally associated with stretch reflex activity in the limb muscles maintaining body posture, it has recently been suggested (Öhman, 1967; MacNeilage, 1970; Hardcastle, 1970; Bowman, 1971) that the spindle has a possible important function in the myodynamic control of speech production, so it will now be described in detail.

To understand the functions of the spindle, it is necessary to outline in some detail its morphological structure. Because of its extreme complexity, however, it is only possible here to discuss some of the relatively uncontroversial parts of the spindle and their possible functional significance. Most of the following outline is derived from papers delivered at a number of recent symposia on the subject of muscle spindles (Barker, 1962; Granit, 1966; Andrew, 1966) and from several notable reviews on the subject that have been published (Cooper, 1960; Jansen, 1966; Matthews, 1964, 1972; Granit, 1970).

A semidiagrammatic representation of a typical muscle spindle is shown in Fig. 5. Within the connective-tissue sheath of the spindle lie a number of small intrafusal fibres running parallel to the main extrafusal fibres of the muscle. The intrafusal fibres (up to ten in number) are bound together by the sheath which, near the middle of the spindle

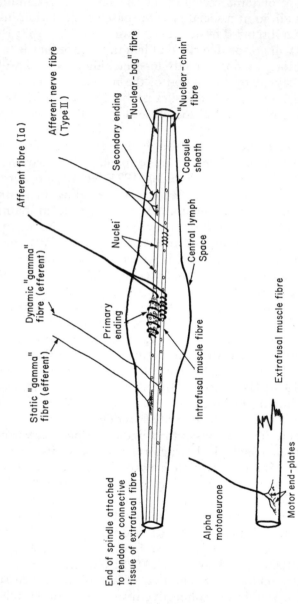

Afferent fibre (Ia)

Afferent nerve fibre (Type II)

Secondary ending

"Nuclear-bag" fibre

"Nuclear-chain" fibre

Capsule sheath

Central lymph Space

Intrafusal muscle fibre

Nuclei

Primary ending

Dynamic "gamma" fibre (efferent)

Static "gamma" fibre (efferent)

End of spindle attached to tendon or connective tissue of extrafusal fibre.

Extrafusal muscle fibre

Alpha motoneurone

Motor end-plates

Fig. 5 Parts of a typical muscle spindle (after Boyd, 1962).

bulges out in a small swelling containing a lymph space. There seems to be general agreement now that most spindles contain two types of intrafusal fibres distinguished by the arrangement of their nuclei in the central lymph space. In fibres of one type, called nuclear-bag fibres, there is an aggregation of nucleii packed closely together. In fibres of the second type, called nuclear-chain fibres, the nucleii are arranged in single file as shown in Fig. 5 (Boyd, 1962).

Intimately connected to the intrafusal fibres are two types of receptors called the primary and secondary endings. Each spindle has one and only one primary ending; it may, however, have a number of secondary endings. The primary ending consists of spirals around the central parts of both the nuclear-bag and nuclear-chain fibres and has a large diameter afferent fibre (type Ia) with high conduction velocity, comparable in size with the alpha motoneurones; this makes them probably larger than the sensory fibres supplying other mechano-receptors, e.g. those responding to touch and pressure. Because of its histological shape, the primary ending is often referred to as an annulo-spiral ending. Secondary endings lie mainly on nuclear-chain fibres (Roberts, 1966, p. 71) although Boyd has them connected to the nuclear-bag fibres as well. They usually take the form of sprays of fine fibre branches sending their impulses via smaller, type IIa fibres.

Because of the anatomical arrangement of the primary endings and the structure of the central part of the spindle, their receptors respond both to the degree of stretch of the central, non-contractile part of the spindle and to the rate of change of stretch as well. The response to maintained stretch, the static response, increases approximately linearly with the length of the muscle. The response to velocity of stretch is called the dynamic response and increases in proportion to the rate of change of muscle length. These two components of primary ending response, the static and dynamic, may have important functions in the control of speech production (see Section IV. B). As far as secondary endings are concerned, it seems likely that they are much less sensitive to velocity of stretch than the primary endings. To static extension, however, the firing frequency is comparable with that of the primary endings, increasing approximately linearly with muscle length. The precise function of the secondary endings is a little uncertain at the present time so they will not be discussed in any great detail here.

Primary endings, therefore, respond to both degree of stretch and velocity of stretch of the central part of the spindle. Investigations on the spinal nerves (Liddell and Sherrington, 1925) have shown that the primary afferent fibres of the spindle make direct synaptic connections with motoneurones to the muscle in which the spindle is situated. Thus any activity in the large type I afferent fibres from primary endings may result in a direct firing of the main alpha motoneurones to the extrafusal fibres causing the muscle to contract. This mechanism is the basis of the so-called stretch reflex loop which can be seen clearly in its rudimentary form in the familiar knee jerk. Figure 6 shows a typical diagram of a stretch reflex loop in the spinal system. It is probable that a similar mechanism occurs in the cranial nerve system with the spindle

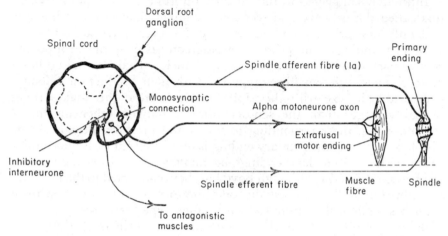

Fig. 6 A basic stretch reflex loop showing the monosynaptic connection between the type Ia afferent fibre from the spindle and the alpha motoneurone to the extrafusal muscle fibre.

afferent fibres from articulatory muscles, although it is undoubtedly more complex.

Now stretch on the central part of the muscle spindle, which causes the firing in the afferent fibres, can be brought about in a number of ways; either as a result of lengthening of the main extrafusal fibres to which the spindle is attached (see Fig. 5) or as a result of contraction of the intrafusal fibres within the spindle, usually by means of the spindle efferent (gamma) fibres.

If the muscle is lengthened, the increasing firing of the primary afferent fibres will reflexly increase activity of the motoneurones to the extrafusal fibres of that muscle because of the monosynaptic connections (see Fig. 6). Thus lengthening of the muscle may be opposed by contraction, and a state of equilibrium will be achieved. If the contraction of antagonistic muscles (or whatever it is that is causing the muscle lengthening) is relaxed, discharge of the primary ending will decrease rapidly, so diminishing the effect of the stretch reflex loop. Because of this reflex activity, the primary afferent and alpha motor system is said to constitute a servo-system with obvious importance, for instance, in maintaining body posture against the opposing force of gravity. This reflex activity is said to take place in the lower co-ordinating centres of the brain, probably the cerebellum, so is a largely automatic activity (Matthews, 1964; Bowman, 1971, pp. 106–108). Also, because the primary impulses are sent via large diameter afferent fibres, which have high conduction velocity, and probably make monosynaptic connections with the motoneurones, the reflex loop will be extremely fast acting. This rapidity may be important for controlling fast movements required for speech production.

The other means by which stretch can be exerted on the central part of the spindle is by the contraction of intrafusal fibres. Originally, this was thought to result from firing of small gamma motoneurones only (see Section II.D.1). It seems now, however, that for some spindles at least, the intrafusal fibres may also be innervated by collaterals of large alpha motoneurones which supply the ordinary extrafusal fibres (Bessou et al., 1965). The functional significance of this alpha innervation and its relevance for spindle control in humans is difficult to assess in the light of present knowledge. Far more information is needed about the frequency of occurrence of this alpha innervation in different muscles. The picture is further complicated by the presence of at least two types of gamma efferent fibres distinguished by their effects on the primary ending discharge. Dynamic gamma fibres increase the dynamic sensitivity of primary endings, i.e. their response to velocity of stretch, whereas static gamma fibres diminish the dynamic sensitivity. Both types excite the receptors in a similar way at constant muscle length. Some investigators (Roberts, 1966, p. 70) have observed that dynamic gammas are responsible mainly for innervating the nuclear-chain fibres and static gammas innervate the nuclear-bag fibres, although both types of fibres may sometimes occur in both types of intrafusal fibres.

There is general agreement now among physiologists that the higher parts of the nervous system (e.g. the motor cortex) can control gamma motoneurones independently of the alpha motoneurones and that they also exert separate control over the gamma motoneurones of different muscles (Matthews, 1964, p. 270). Also, because of the anatomical separation of the static and dynamic gammas, it seems likely that these are separately controlled as well. The ability of the CNS to exert independent control over these different types of fusimotor (i.e. spindle efferent) fibres may have important implications for the co-ordination of muscular activity, which will be discussed later.

It can be seen from the above outline, that activity of the fusimotor fibres reflexly causes firing in the main alpha motoneurones and so muscular contraction (see Fig. 6). Some investigators (Kuffler and Hunt, 1952) have suggested that the importance of fusimotor fibres is to maintain the afferent flow from spindles in spite of a certain amount of mechanical shortening of the spindle (Matthews, 1964, p. 274). It was shown earlier how primary ending discharges decreased rapidly if stretch on the muscle was relaxed suddenly. If, however, fusimotor control were maintained, the sensory and reflex functions of the spindle could be preserved during the rapid shortening.

An alternative suggestion which, because of its considerable theoretical importance in the myodynamic control of speech has attracted widespread attention, is that the muscle spindles and fusimotor fibres form part of a "follow-up length servo" by means of which a muscle can be reflexly set to any desired length. The suggestion was originally formulated by Merton (1953) and has since been discussed at length by a number of different investigators in physiology (Roberts, 1966; Rushworth, 1969; Bowman, 1971, pp. 43–45) and in phonetics (Öhman, 1967; MacNeilage, 1970).

The basic argument involves the operation of the stretch reflex loop discussed above. It was seen how, by reflexly opposing lengthening of the muscle by contraction, the stretch reflex acted like a servo-system (see Fig. 6), thus maintaining the muscle at a fixed length only. Fusimotor discharge provides one way in which the muscle can be set reflexly to a variety of lengths. Any increase in fusimotor activity will cause a corresponding increase in the frequency of discharge from the primary endings, and this will reflexly cause the muscle to shorten until the discharge of the primary ending is reduced to its previous value. (Primary ending discharge decreases, of course, with muscular contraction both in the presence and absence of fusimotor activity.) Thus, if a fusimotor command is sent appropriate to the desired length of the muscle, this length will be automatically achieved irrespective of the length of the muscle at the beginning of the movement. This principle has been specifically suggested by a number of investigators as one of the possible means of solving the problem of motor equivalence (Milner, 1967, 1970; MacNeilage, 1970), i.e. the fact that we almost never perform an act such as an articulatory movement, exactly the same way twice; there are always minor or major variations on the movements made, depending on local conditions at the time, etc. As Milner (1970, p. 67) says

"Input instructions determine the result independently of conditions at the specific muscles involved. The servomechanism allows this achievement without requiring storage of an impossibly large number of alternative sets of instructions at the higher levels."

The local conditions may include not only the tension and length of the muscle before the movement but changes in tension, etc. as a result of some external force during the movement. Compensation for any external force will take place by means of the stretch reflex servo-system.

In this view, therefore, the fusimotor fibres are seen as a pathway for initiating movements, by their effects on the muscle spindles rather than as a compensation for the effects of movement upon the spindle. There is some evidence to suggest that discharge of gamma motoneurones may precede that of alpha motoneurones in the same muscle (Cooper, 1960, p. 412; Matthews, 1964, p. 275) but this is by no means conclusively established. It seems reasonable to assume that for any voluntary movement, e.g. a particular speech articulation, sufficient gamma and alpha activity is sent appropriate to the target position and velocity of movement. As Matthews (1964, p. 277) says,

> "The alpha route would perhaps be most efficiently employed in conjunction with sufficient fusimotor activity to prevent any decrease in spindle discharge occurring during the contraction; this would be achieved if the relative amounts of alpha and gamma activity were adjusted to be appropriate for the velocity of shortening 'expected' under any particular set of conditions. Then if shortening proceeded faster than 'intended' by the higher centres it would be slowed by servo action and if shortening were hindered by some unexpected load it would be speeded up by servo action".

The spindle thus can perhaps be regarded as playing a dual role in not only providing moment-to-moment information on the degree of tension and rate of change of tension in the muscle, but also acting as an essential element in a servo-mechanism system by means of the stretch reflex loop.

## 1. Distribution of Sensory Resources in the Oral Region

Some recent histological studies (Cooper, 1953; Grossman, 1964; Dixon, 1962) have indicated that the sensory receptors mentioned in the previous section are not evenly distributed throughout the oral region. After a review of the histological literature relating to tactile receptors in the oral mucosa, Grossman (1964, p. 132) concludes that there is a progressive decrease in the frequency of sensory endings from the front to the rear of the mouth in humans. This progression is particularly noticeable in the tongue, where the tip seems better endowed with sensory receptors subserving tactile and pressure sensations than any other part of the oral system (Grossman and Hattis, 1967). It is interesting to note also that this progression seems to apply to the oral tissues of other species as well (Kamada, 1955).

Research by Cooper (1953) suggests also that there is a differential distribution of muscle spindles in the tongue. She found most spindles in the superior longitudinalis muscle near the mid-line and in the front third of the tongue, and in the transversus muscle in the mid-region towards the lateral borders. It is significant that a relatively greater density of muscle spindles has been found in those parts of the muscles which are plausibly thought of as needing the maximum delicacy of adjustment in the production of complex articulations such as [s], [ʃ], etc.

The relatively large number and variety of sensory receptors particularly the tactile receptors of both diffuse and organized types in the anterior part of the tongue, suggests that this part of the organ is capable of a considerable range of sensory discriminations, many of which are probably important for the control of speech production. The delicacy of tactile sensory discriminations in the front of the mouth is well illustrated by two-point discrimination tests (Ringel and Ewanowski, 1965) which show an increasing degree of tactile acuity towards the lips. In addition, oral stereognosis studies (Bosma, 1967) have shown that the anterior two-thirds of the tongue is primarily important in oral discriminations probably involving an integration of both tactile and proprioceptive (i.e. muscle spindle and joint) receptors. It is interesting to note in this regard that Penfield and Boldrey (1937) noted frequent responses involving the front of the tongue and lips after electrical stimulation of the cortex, but relatively infrequent responses in the back of the tongue. It is interesting also that articulations such as [s] and [ʃ] involving maximally complex movements and configurations of the tongue, and consequently, relatively delicate control by the various sensory receptor feedback systems, are more likely to occur in the anterior part of the mouth than in the back part. The relatively rich supply of sensory resources in the anterior oral region makes such delicate control possible.

## IV.  Sensori-Motor Co-ordination

### A.   Importance of Sensory Feedback Control of Speech Production

So far in this chapter it has been shown how the motor system transmits neural impulses to the muscles from the CNS and how the receptor organs at the periphery of the body or within muscles send "back" via the afferent nerves, different sorts of information about the characteristics of the stimuli applied to them. It remains to be shown how in fact the CNS makes use of this sensory system to co-ordinate movements. The importance of sensory feedback for motor co-ordination has not always been recognized. Early research workers believed there was a one-to-one relationship between discrete chains of motor impulses from the CNS and equally discrete movements at the periphery. As Bernstein (1967, p. 145) notes,

> "Physiologists of the last century (e.g. Munk, Bekhterev) saw the motor area of the cortex as a sort of keyboard on which somebody's hand, in sovereign control, described the program for a given motor stereotype. The pressing (excitation) of one of these cell buttons always brought about a given degree of flexion at a given joint, the pressing of a second brought about extension, etc."

This is, of course, far too simplistic a view of the operation of the nervous system; it does not take account of the multiplicity of motor patterns depending on the state of the muscle at any given time, due to external forces such as gravity, friction, etc., or of the complex neural pathways involving many synapses (see above Section II.C).

It is quite clear now that the only way motor co-ordination is possible is by constant sensory feedback from receptors at the periphery. As Bernstein (1967, pp. 106–107) puts it,

> "The motor effect of a central impulse cannot be decided at the centre but is decided entirely at the periphery; at the last spinal and myoneural synapse, at the muscle, in the mechanical and anatomical changes of force in the limb being moved, etc. The central effectors achieve co-ordination of movements only by plastically reacting to the totality of the signals from the afferent field, adapting the impulses transmitted to the situation that actually obtains at the periphery."

It was indicated above how sensory resources provide the CNS with continuous information on the position, acceleration and velocity of the vocal organs in terms of trains of neural impulses. It is conceivable that the CNS integrates reports from different receptors and receptor-types to give a dynamic *schema* or running plot of the state of the vocal organs. (Cf. the body *schema* of Head and Holmes (1920), which they describe as an unconscious physiological record of the body posture.) There are two ways in which the CNS probably makes use of information of this dynamic *schema* type: by means of such systems as reflex mechanisms (for instance, stretch reflex loops), and by comparing the running plot of an actual articulation with the running plot of sensory information that the brain would expect from successful execution of the normal appropriate articulation. If these two *schemata* do not match the brain may formulate an appropriate compensatory program.

Exactly how these complex integration processes are carried out in the CNS is not yet fully understood. A closer look at the feedback systems and their possible function in speech articulation may, however, throw some light on this problem.

## B. Different Types of Feedback used in Speech Articulation

Two main types of sensory feedback circuits, the exteroceptive and proprioceptive, are probably used for the myodynamic control of speech. The exteroceptive circuits include auditory feedback, reporting on bone and air conduction of vibratory and acoustic stimuli in the ear, and tactile feedback reporting on contacts between different vocal organs, for example the tongue against the palate. The proprioceptive circuits report on the tension of the muscles and movements of the joints.

### 1. The Auditory System

The sensory receptors in the auditory feedback system are specialized mechanoreceptors situated in the Organ of Corti, which is a complex structure occupying the length and breadth of the basilar membrane in the inner ear. The receptors, which take the form of tiny hair cells, respond to movement of the basilar membrane by sending trains of neural impulses through their respective nerve fibres. This movement of the basilar membrane directly reflects the vibration produced by sound waves striking the ear-drum.

Information concerning the frequency, intensity, duration and tonal qualities of the sound wave is sent from the receptor organs through the vestibulo-cochlear (VIII cranial) nerce to be projected finally on the "auditory" cortex (Zemlin, 1968). The so-called volley–place theory proposed by Wever (1949) describes how information concerning the frequency and intensity of a sound can be sent via the acoustic nerve fibres. According to this theory there are two mechanisms for coding and transmitting information on the frequency of the stimulus. Low frequency sounds are discriminated by volleys of nerve impulses in the acoustic nerve fibres, which reflect the stimulus frequency. High frequency sounds, however, are mediated on the basis of the place on the basilar membrane where maximum stimulation occurs. Increased intensity of the stimulus is reflected mainly in firing rates of individual nerve fibres, without affecting the composite pattern frequency for a particular pitch.

So far we have discussed the auditory feedback channel as involving transmission of sound waves through the air which impinge upon the ear-drum. Another avenue by which we hear sounds, however, is by bone conduction. Bone conduction of sound occurs when various parts of the skull vibrate during speech so activating the inner ear in much the same way as sound conduction.

Because it involves transmission of sound through the air or bone, feedback of information through the auditory channel is necessarily slower than through the tactile or proprioceptive channels. Auditory feedback only operates after the event, for example after the articulation of a particular vowel.

## 2. The Tactile System

The receptors in the tactile circuit include the free endings and organized endings discussed in the first part of Section III.B. Most of the sensory fibres from the tactile receptors in the oral region are contained in the trigeminal, vagus and glossopharyngeal cranial nerves, making many synaptic connections with other neurones before finally being projected in the somesthetic cortex in certain specific areas corresponding to positions of the body (Penfield and Rasmussen, 1950). In addition to their cerebro-cortical projection most afferent fibres from the oral region project onto the cerebellum. This is presumably to aid the cerebellum in its co-ordinatory and monitoring function. The calibre size of the fibres from the tactile receptors are in general smaller than those from the primary endings of muscle spindles so their conduction velocity is slightly less.

How in fact the CNS integrates all the sensory data arriving from such receptors is an extremely complex problem. However, some of the principles of neural circuits such as spatial summation at synaptic junctions, that were discussed earlier (see Section II.C) suggest how this complex integration may be carried out.

It was seen earlier how each nerve cell in the nervous system receives impulses from many other cells. To take a simple example, suppose a group of neurones, A, receive impulses from say, free endings in the tongue tip and another group of neurones, B, receive impulses from Meissner corpuscles and other pressure receptors. Now an interneurone C, may receive in turn impulses from both group A and group B. If pressure is applied to the tongue tip, for example in the articulation of an alveolar stop, there will be an increased chance of firing occurring in neurones of group A and also in neurones of group B. Correspondingly, there will be increased chance of firing of interneurone C, because of the principle of spatial summation. In this situation therefore we could infer that activity of the interneurone C had been preceded by the presentation of a pressure stimulus to the tip of the tongue.

Although this is, of course, an extremely over-simplified case, it may be possible, proceeding along similar lines, to theoretically map out pathways for physiological messages through the CNS without relying at any stage on a one-to-one synapse with guaranteed transmission. These pathways may provide the physiological basis for the dynamic *schema* outlined in the previous section.

As was seen earlier, the physiological characteristics of the tactile receptor systems enable information to be sent to the CNS concerning localization of contact, degree of deformation of the oral surfaces, and the onset time of contact. Thus the feedback of information through the tactile channel takes place after the event, e.g. after contact occurs between the tongue and alveolar region of the palate during the occlusion phase in the production of an alveolar stop. The proprioceptive feedback system, on the other hand, can transmit information concerning muscular activity during an event.

## 3. The Proprioceptive System

The receptor organs contributing to vocal proprioceptive feedback are the muscle spindles, joint receptors, and special endings called Golgi tendon organs. These latter organs are receptors attached to the tendons of muscles. They respond to stretch on the tendon, and their main purpose is probably to act as "safety valves" inhibiting the muscle when too much tension is exerted (cf. Cooper, 1960, p. 416).

Some aspects of the anatomy and physiology of muscle spindles have been outlined in Section III.B. It was seen how fusimotor activity, originating in the cortex, may play an important role in the myodynamic control of speech by setting a muscle reflexly to attain a specific length irrespective of local conditions of the muscle prevailing at any given time. This system provides a very powerful means by which, for instance, a target configuration appropriate for an articulation such as [t] will be similar in two different environments such as [a t a] and [i t i], the actual differences being due to such factors as biomechanical constraints of the muscle, external forces acting on the muscle, mutual dependence on context, etc. This target configuration can thus be "set" without continuous motor commands being sent from the higher centres.

It was also suggested earlier, that firing of dynamic fusimotor fibres may have the effect of accelerating the contraction of the muscle as a whole and so assist in attaining, more rapidly, the target configurations required for speech production. This may happen, for instance, in the articulation of [a t a], where the tongue tip has to move a greater distance than for [i t i]. The time taken to move that greater distance, however, may not be longer because of dynamic fusimotor activity enhancing the appropriate extrafusal muscle firing.

It was also suggested earlier that the muscle spindle may play an important part in the reflex control of sensori-motor co-ordination. At an elementary level, reflex mechanisms can be regarded as basic stimulus–response activities. Stimulus in the form of stretch on the primary ending of the spindle causes a sensory discharge, which in turn causes the muscle to contract. Such mechanisms usually occur below the level of the cortex; they are, as Di Salvo (1961, p. 336) notes,

"Very efficient and purposeful types of mechanisms, whereby lower levels of the CNS may control functions which satisfy basic needs, leaving higher levels of the brain free to subserve behaviour of a more optional kind."

Primary ending discharge probably plays an important part in providing information about muscle activity appropriate to the *schemata* of different articulations, particularly during a movement. Because of the probable direct monosynaptic pathway of the reflex loop and the fact that the impulses travel in large, high conduction velocity fibres, this type of feedback mechanism is extremely fast acting (Milner, 1970, p. 73). This rapidity may be important for sensori-motor control of speech where many different muscular activities take place every second. It is possible also that the muscle spindle system may provide the CNS with "predictive" information about muscle activity. This is made possible by the response of the primary endings to rate of change in muscle length thus enabling the CNS to compute the probable length a muscle may achieve after a given period of time.

In addition to the monosynaptic connections with the motoneurones of its muscles, the afferent fibres of the spindle also have polysynaptic connections with inhibitory and excitatory neurones (see Section II.C), whereby the primary discharges not only help to activate the original muscle but to activate also synergistic muscles and inhibit the antagonists (Cooper, 1960, p. 413). For an articulation such as [s] (which will be used throughout this book as an example of a characteristically complex articulation), requiring finely graded control of both protagonist and antagonist muscles, the ratio of excitatory to inhibitory discharges is probably appropriately different.

It was mentioned above that the trigeminal nerve was responsible for providing tactile feedback from the anterior two-thirds of the tongue. It is by no means certain, however, that this nerve also provides the afferent innervation for the muscle spindles. Many investigators have suggested that the hypoglossal or twelfth cranial nerve originally thought to be a purely motor nerve, has a sensory component along which impulses may travel from the spindles (Langworthy, 1924; Tarkhan, 1936; Bowman, 1971; Adatia and Gehring, 1971), although this opinion is not shared by all. Barron (1936) thought that proprioceptive impulses from the tongue musculature are conducted by the lingual nerve, part of the trigeminal (cranial nerve V) system.

The fact that the autonomic component is intimately mixed in some cranial nerves makes the situation more confused. This, and other factors have severely hampered research into the sensory innervation of striated muscles in the territory of the cranial nerves (Hosokawa, 1961, p. 405).

The table on pp. 32, 33 is a summary of the main features of the three main feedback systems used in the control of speech production. It should not be assumed that these are the only feedback systems available: there are probably other similar systems utilizing different types of receptor organs in the vocal organs, which have yet to be investigated.


## C. Relative Importance of Different Types of Feedback in Speech Articulation

Some investigators consider some types of feedback more important than others for the purposes of speech. Thus Fry (1957) states that "by far the most important" feedback loop is the auditory, followed by kinesthetic (equivalent to proprioceptive in this context) feedback, with tactile feedback not seeming to play an important role at all. Various investigators since (Ringel and Steer, 1963; Ladefoged, 1967), however, have questioned the primacy of auditory feedback.

The role of the different feedback systems in speech production has usually been investigated in two different types of experiments. One type involves studying the speech output of patients with various identifiable somesthetic abnormalities (MacNeilage et al., 1967), and the other involves experimentally altering normal sensory feedback, usually by interfering with the functioning of the relevant receptor organs, and examining the effects of such alteration on speech production

(McCroskey, 1958; Ringel and Steer, 1963; Ladefoged, 1967; Schliesser and Coleman, 1968; Weiss, 1969; Gammon *et al.*, 1971; Scott and Ringel, 1971; Hardcastle, 1975). Methods used to experimentally alter tactile sensory receptor functioning include various types of local anaesthetics, which can be applied directly onto the surface of the oral mucosa or injected into the mandibular branch of the trigeminal nerve, which supplies sensory reception for a large part of the oral region, including the front two-thirds of the tongue. Normal functioning of the auditory feedback channel can be altered by the application of high-amplitude masking noise. Most of these studies indicated that interference with tactile feedback channels caused significant alterations in articulation, particularly the achievement of target positions for complex sounds such as [s] and [ʃ]. Auditory masking was found generally to cause alterations in vocal intensity, intraoral air pressure, duration of articulation and fundamental frequency.

The results of these experiments indicate that rather than one type of feedback being more important than another for speech in general, it is probably more true to say that the exploitation of a given type of sensory feedback may vary in its importance depending on the category of articulation involved. Thus articulations involving contact between articulatory organs such as alveolar stops, etc., may utilize fully the tactile resources, while articulations involving no contact, for example, low back vowels, may utilize maximally the auditory and probably also the proprioceptive feedback channels.

## 1. Role of Sensory Resources in Anticipatory "Tuning in Advance"

It was seen earlier that for the nervous system to make full use of the different types of feedback mechanisms for speech, they must be efficient and fast-acting so that the speaker can continuously check the accuracy of the execution of the intended articulation. If any discrepancy occurs between the intended articulation and that which actually takes place, a monitoring system may correct the myodynamic performance. This probably happens for instance in the detection and correction of slips of the tongue (Laver, 1969).

This monitoring process may be facilitated by "priming in advance" not only the execution of motor actions but also the exteroceptive and proprioceptive "expectations" appropriate to these actions. As far as execution of motor actions is concerned, it is probable that for skilled, rapid muscular activities such as those required for speech, the neural correlates of these actions are "primed" or "pre-set" before the performance of the utterance begins (Lashley, 1951). Evidence of this can

|  | Tactile | Proprioceptive | Auditory |
|---|---|---|---|
| Type of sensory receptors | A. free endings<br>B. complex endings (e.g. Krause end-bulbs, Meissner corpuscles). | A. muscle spindles<br>B. Golgi tendon organs<br>C. joint receptors | A. haircells in Organ of Corti |
| Distribution of receptors | A. epithelium, connective tissue between papillae<br>B. lamina propria, particularly deeper layers in oral region | A. all speech muscles<br>B. tendons<br>C. capsules of joints | A. Organ of Corti throughout length and breadth of basilar membrane |
| Information sent to the CNS | A 1. localization of contact<br>+ 2. pressure of contact<br>B 3. direction of movement<br>4. onset time of contact | A 1. length of muscle fibre<br>2. degree of stretch of fibre<br>3. velocity of stretch<br>4. direction of movement of muscle<br>B 1. change of stretch on tendon by muscular contraction, etc.<br>C 1. rate of joint movement<br>2. direction of joint movement<br>3. extent of movement | 1. intensity<br>2. frequency<br>3. duration<br>4. tonal qualities |

| Main feature of the feedback system | | | |
|---|---|---|---|
| | 1. slower acting than proprioceptive because<br>(a) multisynaptic pathway<br>(b) afferent fibres smaller<br>2. spatial projection of peripheral receptive surface preserved in sensory cortex<br>3. probably transmits information *after* the event<br>4. important for speech movements involving contact between articulators, e.g. [t], [i], etc. | 1. fast acting because<br>(a) monosynaptic<br>(b) spindle afferent fibres largest in body<br>2. predictive information important for servo operation<br>3. speech target invariance by means of follow-up length servo operation of gamma loop system<br>4. provides information *during* the event<br>5. important for all articulations | 1. slower acting than tactile and proprioceptive because transmission of sound through air (for air conduction)<br>2. projection on auditory cortex preserves spatial characteristics of basilar membrane, also projections to other areas<br>3. supplies information *after* the event<br>4. important for open and back vowels, e.g. [a], [o], etc. |

be found in anticipatory tongue slips (Boomer and Laver, 1968) and in co-articulation phenomena (Öhman, 1966, 1967; Daniloff and Moll, 1968; MacNeilage and De Clerk, 1969; Daniloff and Hammarberg, 1973). Lashley (1951, p. 188), when speaking of the pre-set mechanism referred particularly to a certain type of fast accurate movement such as a whip-cracking motion with the hand, which, he claimed, could not be continuously monitored by sensory feedback from higher levels, because

> "the entire movement from initiation to completion requires less than the reaction time for tactile and kinesthetic stimulation . . ."

It is conceivable, however, that the neural correlates of sensory resources may be primed in advance or tuned in in much the same way as motor execution is. As Bernstein (1967, p. 162) says,

> "proceeding with a determined program of operation, the central nervous system can, and indeed does, achieve anticipatory adaption in terms of the tuning in advance of the arousal of all the sensory and motor elements which are employed . . ."

Such anticipatory tuning in advance may not only facilitate the monitoring process but may also be a means by which on-going sensory feedback control is facilitated.

Ongoing or "closed-loop" sensory feedback control may also be facilitated by the "predictive" function of the muscle spindles mentioned above. This enables the CNS to maintain control during a movement without waiting for sensory information to be sent back through the exteroceptive circuits after completion of the movement.

# 2

# Biomechanical Constraints on Muscular Activity

## I. Introductory

In Chapter 1 it was seen how muscles are innervated by peripheral neural elements and how sensory components probably contribute to the feedback control of motor activity. Most of the examples given considered the activity of a single muscle or single receptor organ. In reality, of course, any voluntary movement requires the co-ordinated activity of many different muscles, some being excited while others are inhibited, with probably thousands of receptor organs reporting on different aspects of the movement. It is important to realize that the actual mechanical activity of muscles, their contracting and relaxing, is automatic, in that their activity is entirely subject to neural signals; it is the CNS that is responsible for the achievement of any voluntary movement. Thus the CNS probably initiates a "plan" of the spatio-temporal aspects of the movement or series of movements, the details of which may be sorted out at a sub-cortical level, partly under the influence of sensory feedback from the organs concerned.

Thus it is possible that contraction of a particular muscle will usually be accompanied by a compensatory relaxation of its antagonist and vice versa, the extent of contraction being automatically determined by sensory feedback, particularly proprioceptive feedback, depending on prevailing conditions at any given time. Some articulations, however, particularly those requiring delicately controlled tongue configurations require a "balanced" contraction of both protagonist and antagonist muscles.

As muscular contraction is the basis of all speech movement it is important to consider biomechanical constraints of the muscle, which will affect the course of the activity. In the discussion on motor units it was seen how the time taken by a muscle to reach peak tension depends to some extent on the frequency at which the successive activations follow one another in each motor unit. It was also seen how the tension developed by a muscle depends on the number of motor units active at any given time. As the tension increases, more and more motor units are activated. It remains to be shown how the force developed by a muscle can also depend on inherent properties in the muscle itself.

## II. Mechanics of Muscular Contraction

How does a voluntary muscle in fact produce the mechanical effect of contraction? To answer this question it is necessary to consider the microstructure of the muscle fibres themselves. Recently, electron microscopy studies (Huxley, 1965, 1969; Bourne, 1972, pp. 302–388) have shown that striated muscle fibres consist of longitudinally orientated myofibrils, arranged so that the fibre has an appearance of being divided into transverse bands (hence the name striated muscle). The striations divide the myofibrils into structural sub-units called sarcomeres within which there is an orderly array of two types of protein filaments, actin and myosin. Contraction of the muscle is caused by the sliding of actin filaments between myosin filaments while the lengths of the individual filaments remain unaltered. This mechanism also means that the filaments and so the fibres, are not distorted during contraction. Where the myosin and actin filaments overlap, cross-bridges (Huxley, 1965, p. 10) are formed; the tension developed by muscle fibres being related to the number of cross-bridges. Hypotheses concerning the means by which electrical potentials arriving via the motoneurones are transformed into mechanical work in sliding filaments past each other, have been put forward by a number of investigators (Huxley, 1969) and will not be discussed here.

The main force-developing component of the muscle therefore corresponds to the actin/myosin complex described above, which may vary from muscle to muscle (Szent-Györgyi, 1953). The sarcome reorganization within a muscle will determine, for instance, the relationship between the load a muscle has to move and the maximal velocity at which the load can be moved. In general the lighter the duty, the swifter the movement (Gelfan, 1955, pp. 134–135; Cunningham, 1964, p. 268). Most of the speech muscles particularly the muscles of the tongue need to have steep tension/velocity curves to enable them to achieve the rapid movements involved in speech production.

Not only the microstructure of a muscle, but also the arrangement of the muscle fibres themselves, and their manner of attachment to tendons and other elastic tissue material, will have some influence on the tension characteristics of the muscle as a whole. Among the speech muscles, there are three main types of muscle structure: parallel, fan-like and pennate. The parallel type consists of muscle fibres running parallel with the length of the muscle. In general a long slender parallel muscle (e.g. stylohyoideus) has little power but can shorten through a relatively large distance (up to 50%). A short broad muscle (e.g. intercostals) on the other hand can contract with considerable force but through a very short distance. Fan-like muscles (e.g. temporalis) consist of fibres which converge onto a single tendon from a relatively broad origin. They have a short range of motion but can exert great power. This power is important in muscles like the temporalis, one of the primary functions of which is to grind the back teeth together in mastication. Pennate fibres (such as in the mylohyoideus) are shaped like a feather with the fibres converging onto a central raphe. Like the fan type, pennate muscles are relatively powerful but have a small range of motion.

## III. General Problems of Co-ordination and Timing of Muscular Contractions

### A. Biomechanical Constraints on Muscular Activity

In addition to the force-developing component of muscle (the actin/myosin complex) described in the previous section, there is also an elastic component, which will considerably influence the force a muscle can exert. The elastic component consists of connective tissue within the muscle (accounting for about 15% of the total weight of the muscle) and tendons at the ends of muscles if they are attached to bones. As all muscles contain the elastic component, it must be taken into account in assessing the force developed by the muscle and the time taken to achieve peak tension. This is so because lengthening of the elastic component increases the load on the contractile component so reducing the speed of shortening.

Various models have been proposed to estimate the actual time course of events at the contractile machinery (e.g. Hill, 1953). Hill's work and others are reviewed in considerable detail by Davson (1970).

Other factors, such as the mass and inertia of the muscle, the work done against gravity and the mechanical properties of the imposed load must be taken into account in considering muscle activity. In the myo-dynamic control of speech therefore, it may be that factors such as the mass and inertia of the speech muscles and speech organs, properties of the imposed load, gravity, friction, etc. may result in "overshoot" or "undershoot" of the target positions irrespective of the fusimotor control mentioned earlier (cf. Tatham, 1969, p. 35).

To sum up, therefore, the degree of force a muscle can develop and the time taken to achieve this force will depend on the following:

(i)    the elasticity of the muscle—tension/length and tension/velocity curves;
(ii)   the number of motor units active at any one time;
(iii)  the frequency of successive activations within motor units;
(iv)   the inherent mechanical properties of the muscle;
(v)    the mechanical properties of the imposed load.


## B. Co-ordination of Muscle Groups

Mechanical activity in a muscle can lead to a number of different effects. These include:

(i)    dynamic shortening of the muscle. In the case of the tongue muscles, contraction may move bones (e.g. the hyoid or mandible), or cause stretch on connecting muscles. This type of contraction is called isotonic contraction;
(ii)   increased tension, where the muscle does not shorten. Such tension changes are called isometric;
(iii)  lengthening. If the opposing force, for instance that exerted by an adjoining muscle is greater than the maximum contraction tension, the muscle is stretched or lengthened while actively contracting.

It can be seen from this that "contraction" has a special meaning referring to changes in mechanical properties. It is a rather unfortunate term because effect (iii) indicates that a muscle can be mechanically active without necessarily shortening.

When a number of muscles function together to achieve a movement of an organ, the various muscles are given different functional names, depending on their role in achieving the overall movement, such as prime movers (or protagonists), antagonists, fixation muscles and synergists. Each of these different roles will be considered in turn.

### a. Prime Movers or Protagonists

These are muscles primarily responsible for effecting the actual movements which occur. When the body of the tongue is moved forward in the mouth the protagonist is the posterior part of the genioglossus muscle. The movement is usually affected by a dynamic shortening of the muscles (i.e. an isotonic movement). When a prime mover contracts it tends to perform all the actions for which it is a mover although some of these actions may be prevented from occurring by other muscles or by external forces.

### b. Antagonists

These muscles may be inhibited from activity during contraction of the protagonists or they may actively contract to oppose the movement. Despite their name, the antagonists can also contract at the same time as the protagonists, contributing to a controlled movement by (Cunningham, 1964, p. 268)

"paying out just as much as and no more than is required, thus securing guidance and precision."

The antagonistic capacity of various muscles is important in achieving delicately controlled tongue configurations such as is necessary in the production of [s].

### c. Fixation Muscles

These provide a stable, fixed base from which other muscles can contract. In achieving many tongue movements, the infrahyoid muscles act as fixation muscles enabling the suprahyoid musculature to exert force on the relatively immobilized hyoid bone.

### d. Synergists

These are usually regarded as muscles assisting the protagonists in effecting a particular movement. The styloglossus can act as a synergist in assisting the intrinsic musculature of the tongue to raise the lateral borders of the tongue for the production of [s].

It is useful, in any organized description of co-ordinated activity such as speech production to outline the main types of movement that can occur as a result of these different kinds of muscular contraction. There are three major types of movement (Rasch and Burke, 1971)— a ballistic movement, a passive movement, or a guided controlled movement. The ballistic movement involves contraction of the prime mover muscle unhindered by antagonists. An example in speech production could be contraction of the posterior genioglossus muscle (with the superior longitudinalis as synergist) raising the front of the tongue for an alveolar tap or stop. A passive movement is one which takes place without continuing muscle contraction. An example would be the torque action of the ribs during passive exhalation (see Chapter 3). A guided controlled movement is necessary in the production of the so-called complex articulations such as [s] and [ʃ] where antagonist activity occurs simultaneously with protagonist to achieve the necessary finely graded configurations of the articulations.

These three types of muscular movement can have important effects on the temporal co-ordination of speech production. It is likely, for example, that a ballistic movement involving primarily protagonist muscular activity will be intrinsically faster than a precisely controlled guided movement involving activity of different muscular groups. This may explain why vowel durations before fricatives are greater than before stops. Stevens and House (1963, p. 126) have postulated on the basis of spectrographic evidence that slower articulator transition movements for fricatives as compared with stops might result from the fact that a greater precision of articulatory control is necessary for fricatives (for example, the narrow grooved configuration for an [s]) than for stops, where any possible "overshoot" arising from the ballistic movement will have a negligible effect on the acoustic signal.

## IV. Special Problems Relating to the Complexities of Timing and Sequence of Muscular Activities during Speech

Lenneberg (1967, p. 91) estimates that the rate at which individual muscular events occur (throughout the speech apparatus) during articulation may be of an order of several hundred events every second. This means that speech probably exploits to co-ordinating systems in the CNS more fully than almost any other volitional activity.

As an example of the problem of temporal integration, one can consider the activity of the tongue musculature in the production of a syllable as apparently simple as [s a t]. Each of the three segments requires a different target position and configuration of the tongue, achieved by balanced contractions involving both the extrinsic and intrinsic tongue muscles. In addition, the position of the mandible and the hyoid bone must be set for each target configuration; this involves utilizing some of the tongue musculature, as well as the hyoid and mandibular musculature. The vocal cords also must be accurately co-ordinated; vibration must begin some time during the release of the [s] in anticipation of the following vowel and must cease during the closure for the final stop. Finally, the respiratory muscles must contract sufficiently to provide energy for the generation of the speech sounds in the form of air-flow through the vocal tract.

In all, probably about thirty-five muscles are directly involved in achieving the articulatory movements and configurations for each segment. When one considers that the three segments represent not three static postutes of the vocal tract, but an almost continuously active sequence of events, where the muscles must contract dynamically in time, the extent of the temporal integration problem can be appreciated.

## V. Methods of Investigating the Physiology of Speech Production

Most of the present knowledge concerning the physiology of speech production comes from three principal sources: anatomical studies, direct and indirect observation of the various articulatory organs in action, and electromyographic investigations. Anatomical information concerning individual muscles associated with various articulatory organs can give valuable clues as to not only the probable direction and extent of movement of the organs but also the temporal constraints on that movement, from knowledge of the inherent properties of the muscle; its size, shape, etc.

In this book the main muscles associated with activity of the speech organs are discussed with reference to their origin, course, insertion, innervation and function. The origin of a muscle is defined as the point where the muscle joins a relatively stationary structure. The course refers to the general direction of the various fibres which make up the muscle. The point of attachment of the muscle onto a relatively moveable part is called the insertion. It frequently happens that the moveable structure is stabilized by fixator muscles so that during muscular contraction, it is the origin not the insertion part that moves. Thus the question as to what is origin and what is insertion often depends on the actual movement itself. For example, the mylohyoideus muscle can contract from a fixed mandible (as origin) to draw the hyoid bone (as insertion) forwards and upwards. However, if the hyoid bone is fixed by the infrahyoid musculature, contraction of the mylohyoideus will retract and lower the mandible. In the latter movement, the hyoid would be regarded as the origin and the mandible as the point of insertion.

The function of a muscle can be inferred from the anatomical details and, where applicable, from the results of electromyographic and other instrumental investigations that have been carried out on that muscle during speech production. The emphasis throughout the book will be on functions of muscles and their contribution to various articulatory movements, so schematic-type diagrams showing probable directions of movement of structures due to muscular contraction, rather than accurate pictorial diagrams are favoured. The use of such diagrams will hopefully serve to illustrate that the speech production mechanism involves the co-ordinated activity of many different muscle groups rather than being primarily concerned with contraction of single muscles. In this respect it will be shown that many muscle groups carry out different functions on different occasions. For example, the suprahyoid muscle group can serve either as depressions of the mandible or as elevators of the larynx (by raising the hyoid bone). Where relevant, such multiple functions of muscle will be pointed out in the course of the following description of the various speech production mechanisms.

# 3
# The Physiology of Respiratory Activity

## I. General Outline of the Skeletal Framework for Respiratory Activity

The activities of speaking and breathing both normally require the production of an airstream in the lungs which is modified in some way by the action of articulatory organs before passing out of the mouth or nose.

The respiratory cycle (i.e. the inhalation and exhalation of air) differs in speaking and breathing: when breathing, the inhalatory part of the cycle is approximately equal in time to the exhalatory part; when speaking, the inhalatory part of the cycle must be very fast and the exhalatory part slowed down.

The exchanges of air during the respiratory cycle are brought about primarily by alterations in the dimensions of the thoracic cavity, which includes the ribs and lungs. When the volume of the thoracic cavity is enlarged, the pressure within the cavity is lowered, and air will be sucked in from the mouth or nose. When, however, the volume of the cavity is decreased, the pressure is raised so forcing air out of the nose or mouth. To understand how these various changes in the dimensions of the thoracic cavity take place, it is necessary firstly to discuss the main anatomical structures forming the skeletal framework of respiratory activity.

Figure 7 shows schematically the main structures involved in respiratory activity. The trachea consists of eighteen connected horseshoe-shaped cartilages, the open ends of which are closed posteriorly by the trachealis muscle. The top of the trachea passes into the larynx while the bottom end divides into twin tubes or bronchi, which pass directly into the lungs. The lungs themselves consist mainly of masses of minute elastic tissue airsacs called alveoli connected by a dense system of tubes. When the volume in the lungs is decreased, air is forced out of these alveoli into the bronchi tubes and out of the trachea. If, however, the lungs are expanded, the alveoli fill with air, which is drawn in from the

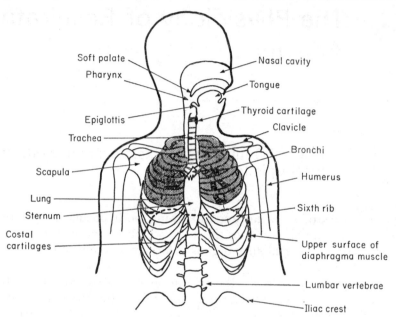

Fig. 7 The arrangement of some of the main structures in the respiratory passage.

trachea due to atmospheric pressure. These changes in the volume of the lungs take place largely by the action of the thoracic cage consisting of the ribs and sternum (or breastbone), and by contraction of the large diaphragma muscle (diaphragm), which separates the lungs from the abdominal cavities.

As Fig. 7 shows, the ribs are twelve in number forming a barrel-shaped protective wall around the thoracic cavity. Posteriorly, the head of each rib is articulated with the vertebral column by means of a special gliding joint. Anteriorly, the first seven ribs join directly onto the sternum by means of costal cartilages, and the next three to a cartilage attached to the lower end of the sternum. The last two ribs (known as floating ribs) have no anterior bony attachments but are fully enveloped in muscle fibres.

Because of the particular shape of the ribs and their anterior and posterior attachments, an upward movement of the ribs will increase the thoracic dimensions in two main planes—the lateral transverse diameter will be increased by virtue of the curved shape of the ribs (particularly the lower ones), while the antero-posterior diameter will be increased by a simultaneous forward and upward movement of the sternum (Rossier *et al.*, 1960).

The vertical dimension of the thoracic cavity can be altered by contraction of the diaphragma muscle. This muscle sits like a dome with its anterior attachments near the sternal connection of the seventh rib (see Fig. 7). When it contracts it presses down on the abdominal viscera and so increases the vertical thoracic dimension. Because of its relatively great strength and speed of contraction, the diaphragma is generally regarded to be the most important muscle for inhalation.

The thoracic framework for breathing is completed by two bones, the clavicle (or collar bone) and scapula (see Fig. 7) which together form the pectoral girdle. The clavicle is articulated medially with the upper surfaces of the sternum and projects laterally to form the main part of the shoulder. The triangular-shaped scapula is attached to the clavicle posteriorly and is covered on both surfaces by muscles. It lies just lateral to the vertebral column on the posterior–superior wall of the rib cage. The importance of the pectoral girdle for speech lies in the fact that a number of neck and shoulder muscles, which help to raise the thoracic cage, have their points of attachment there.

## II. Physiology of Movements Associated with Inhalation and Exhalation

The main movements of the thoracic cavity during inhalation and exhalation involve the ribs and diaphragma muscle. As was indicated in Section I, during inhalation the ribs and sternum are raised, thus decreasing the intrapulmonic pressure. In addition, the vertical dimension of the thoracic cavity is increased by contraction of the diaphragma. For normal speech, the enlargement of the thoracic cavity is brought about mainly by the so-called thoracic muscles, but during emphatic speech many other muscles, for example neck, shoulder and back muscles, can act synergistically. During normal quiet exhalation, elastic recoil forces of muscular tendons, viscera, torque of the ribs, etc.

help to decrease the volume of the thoracic cavity independently of any muscular contraction. However, forced exhalation such as during stressed syllables requires the contribution of thoracic muscles which depress the ribs, and abdominal muscles which compress the abdominal cavity, thus forcing the diaphragma upwards.

According to Draper *et al.* (1960, p. 1843), when the relaxation pressure (created by the elastic recoil forces mentioned above) is greater than the sub-glottal pressure required for phonation, it is opposed by contraction of muscles such as the intercostales externi which tend to raise the ribs, thus prolonging the exhalation phase.

The following is a summary of the main respiratory activities and the muscles contributing to these movements. It should be noted that some muscles can be regarded as having either an inspiratory or an expiratory function, depending on whether their point of origin or insertion is fixed. Those muscles in brackets are involved largely in forced exhalation and inhalation such as required during emphatic speech or shouting. Their role in normal conversational speech is probably minimal.

## A. Muscles of Exhalation
### (i.e. those that lower or decrease the thoracic cavity)

1. Thoracic muscles:
   - *a*. intercostales interni (interosseous portion)
   - *b*. subcostales
   - *c*. transversus thoracis
2. Abdominal muscles:
   - *a*. transversus abdominis
   - *b*. obliquus internus abdominis
   - *c*. obliquus externus abdominis
   - *d*. rectus abdominis
3. Back muscles (for forced exhalation):
   - *a*. latissimus dorsi
   - *b*. iliocostalis
   - *c*. serratus posterior inferior
   - *d*. quadratus lumborum

## B. Muscles of Inhalation
### (i.e. those that enlarge or raise the thoracic cavity)

1. Thoracic muscles:
   - *a*. diaphragma
   - *b*. intercostales interni (intercartilaginous part)
   - *c*. intercostales externi

2. Back muscles (for               *a*. serratus posterior superior
    forced inhalation):          *b*. latissimus dorsi (costal fibres)
                                *c*. levatores costarum
                                *d*. ilicostalis cervicis

3. Neck muscles:                 *a*. sternocleidomastoideus
                                *b*. scalenus

4. Pectoral muscles (for         *a*. pectoralis major
    forced inhalation):          *b*. pectoralis minor
                                *c*. serratus anterior
                                *d*. subclavius

## A. Muscles of Exhalation (Those That Lower or Decrease the Thoracic Cavity)

### 1. Thoracic Muscles

#### *a. Intercostales Interni ("Internal Intercostals")*

*General description:* Layers of short fibres situated between the ribs inferior to the intercostales externi. The fibres are deficient near the vertebral column.

*Origin:* Upper border of first eleven costal cartilages and ribs.

*Course:* Obliquely upwards and forwards approximately at right angles to the intercostales externi (see Section II.B.1.*c*). The fibres are thicker anteriorly than posteriorly.

*Insertion:* Edge of costal groove of the rib directly above.

*Innervation:* Spinal intercostal nerves

*Function:* One important function of the muscle is to act synergistically with the intercostales externi in strengthening the intercostal spaces by coupling the ribs together and preventing the intercostal spaces from bulging outwards. By aiding other muscles such as the abdominal muscles when acting from a fixed pelvis, it can also pull down the rib cage. According to Zemlin (1968, p. 91), the interosseous portion of the muscle is responsible for the latter activity.

Electromyographic investigations by Ladefoged (1967, pp. 1–50) and his associates showed an increase in activity of the intercostales interni muscle as the utterance proceeds, particularly upon termination of pressures involved in relaxation. It was suggested that the intercostales interni together with synergistic activity from the abdominal muscles maintain the pulmonary pressure necessary to activate the vocal folds.

Ladefoged (1967, pp. 1–50) also found bursts of intercostal muscle activity associated with certain articulatory segments such as [h] and long vowels, and before the principal stresses of the utterance during connected speech. These results, however, should be interpreted with some caution as the published examples are restricted to a very small corpus only and most of the published material showed activity of a single motor unit which cannot be said to characterize the muscle as a whole (Lebrun, 1966, p. 73).

### b. Subcostales

*General description:* Small muscles, variable in number, which are situated near the angles of the ribs in the same plane as the innermost fibres of the intercostales interni. The muscle fibres are grouped in thin slips, which are best developed in the lower part of the thorax.
*Origin:* Lower part of the inner surface of the ribs near the angles.
*Course:* Parallel to the intercostales interni.
*Insertion:* The edges of the second or third ribs below.
*Innervation:* Intercostal nerves.
*Function:* The main function of the muscle is probably to aid the intercostales interni in pulling down on the ribs. This activity is made possible when the last rib is fixed by the quadratus lumborum muscle (see Section II.A.3).

### c. Transversus Thoracis

*General description:* A thin, fan-shaped muscle situated inferior to the intercostales on the inside front surface of the thoracic cage.
*Origin:* Inner surface of lower part of sternum.
*Course:* The upper fibres course upwards and the lower lateralward, parallel to the transversus abdominis.
*Insertion:* Posterior surface of ribs two to six.
*Innervation:* Intercostal nerves.
*Function:* When acting from a fixed sternum the muscle can pull down on the ribs to which it attaches (see Fig. 8). Arnold (1968) states that it functions with the intercostales and subcostales muscles so tighten the intercostal spaces during both phases of breathing.

## 2. Abdominal Muscles

### a. Transversus Abdominis

*General description:* A large flat muscle shaped like a girdle or corset located on the front and side of the abdomen. It is the deepest of the abdominal muscles.

*Origin:* Complex origin including the inner surfaces of the costal cartilages of the lower six ribs, (interdigitating with fibres of the diaphragma) the lumbodorsal fascia, the anterior half of the iliac crest,

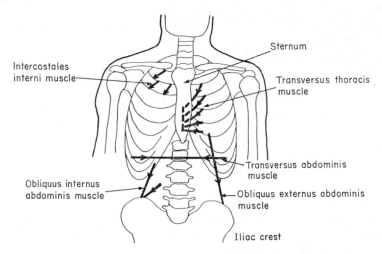

Fig. 8 Some possible directions of movement of the thoracic cage during contraction of some muscles of exhalation. (Intercostales interni muscles extend towards the sternum.)

and the lateral two-thirds of the inguinal ligament (Cunningham, 1972, p. 349 *et seq.*).

*Course:* Horizontal round the abdomen.

*Insertion:* Most fibres attach at the front to the abdominal aponeurosis.

*Innervation:* Intercostal nerves, subcostal, iliohypogastric and ilioinguinal nerves.

*Function:* The main function is to compress the abdomen so raising the abdominal pressure and forcing the diaphragma upwards. This activity decreases the vertical dimension of the thoracic cavity and so aids expiration (see Fig. 8).

### b. Obliquus Internus Abdominis

*General description:* A broad, thin, muscular sheet situated between the obliquus externus and the transversus abdominis muscles.

*Origin:* Anterior half of iliac crest and thorocolumbar fascia.

*Course:* Most fibres run upwards and forwards. Many fibres course forward around the abdomen. The inferior fibres run downward and forward to the pubis.

*Insertion:* The main fibres insert into the abdominal aponeurosis and costal cartilages of the lower three ribs.

*Innervation:* Lower five intercostal, plus iliohypogastric and ilio-inguinal nerves.

*Function:* The main function is to assist the other abdominal muscles in compressing the abdomen thus raising the diaphragma and decreasing the vertical dimension of the thoracic cavity. Also, because of the insertion of some fibres onto the lower three ribs contraction of the muscle may pull down on these ribs (see Fig. 8).

### c. Obliquus Externus Abdominis

*General description:* A flat, broad, superficial muscle covering the surface of the lower thoracic and abdominal wall.

*Origin:* Outer surfaces of lower eight ribs by slips which interdigitate with the serratus anterior and latissimus dorsi muscles (see Sections II.B.4 and II.A.3).

*Course:* Downwards and forwards.

*Insertion:* The lower and posterior fibres insert into the anterior half of the outer lip of the iliac crest. Other fibres insert into the abdominal aponeurosis near the mid-line.

*Innervation:* Lower five intercostal nerves.

*Function:* The main functions are to compress the abdomen and draw the lower ribs downward (see Fig. 8).

### d. Rectus Abdominis

*General description:* A long, flat, strap-like muscle running vertically in the abdominal wall.

*Origin:* Front edge of pubic bone.

*Course:* The fibres travel vertically upwards, widening slightly. Three or more tendinous intersections are attached firmly to the anterior wall of the muscle (Cunningham, 1972, photograph opposite p. 336).

*Insertion:* Anterior surface of the lower part of the sternum and the superficial surfaces of the seventh, sixth and fifth costal cartilages.

*Innervation:* The iliohypogastric and ilio-inguinal nerves, which are branches of the first lumbar nerve innervating some of the muscles of the abdominal wall, and the seventh to twelfth intercostal nerves.

*Function:* The contracting fibres push inwards on the abdominal viscera, so forcing the diaphragma upwards. The muscle can also draw the ribs down by pulling on the sternum. Ladefoged *et al.* (1958, p. 13) noted activity in this muscle only towards the end of a long utterance, thus disagreeing with Stetson (1951, p. 31) who claimed that contraction of the rectus abdominis and other abdominal muscles accompanies each stressed syllable.

## 3. Back Muscles (Only for Forced Exhalation)

### a. Latissimus Dorsi

*General description:* A large, fan-shaped, superficial muscle of the back, whose primary function is to move the arm and shoulder.

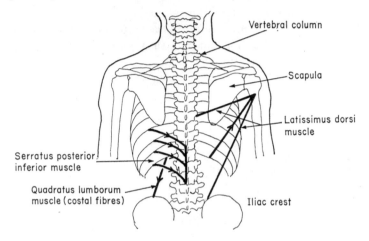

Fig. 9 Back view of the body showing some directions of movement of the thoracic cage during contraction of some muscles of exhalation.

*Origin:* The muscle has a complex origin including the lower portion of the vertebral column and lower ribs, and the iliac crest.
*Course:* The fibres converge as they travel laterally and upward.
*Insertion:* Humerus bone (upper arm).
*Innervation:* Thoracodorsal nerve from the brachial plexus.
*Function:* With the arm fixed, those fibres which are attached to the ribs might lift the ribs and so facilitate inhalation. Contraction of the muscle as a whole, however, is more likely to compress the lower thorax, so aiding exhalation (see Fig. 9). The latissimus dorsi can thus be regarded as a muscle of both inhalation and exhalation.

### b. Iliocostalis

*General description:* One of the deep muscles of the back or vertebral column. There are three main parts to the muscle: lumborum, thoracic

and cervicis. The cervicis is usually regarded as a muscle of inhalation. *Origin:* The lumborum part arises from the lower two lumbar spines, the iliac crest and the sacrum. The thoracic part arises from the lower six ribs medial to the lumborum. The cervicis has its origin on the upper six ribs.
*Course:* All fibres course upwards.
*Insertion:* The lumborum inserts into the lower six ribs, the thoracic into the upper six ribs and the cervicis into the transverse processes of the fourth, fifth, and sixth cervical vertebrae behind the scalenus posterior muscle (see Section II.B.3).
*Innervation:* Posterior rami of spinal nerves.
*Function:* The lumborum and thoracic parts may both function to lower the ribs. In addition the thoracic part may help bind the ribs together. The cervicis may elevate the ribs, and so is regarded as a muscle of inhalation.

### c. Serratus Posterior Inferior

*General description:* A thin, fairly wide back muscle situated on the outer aspect of the lower ribs.
*Origin:* Last two thoracic spinal and first two or three lumbar vertebrae.
*Course:* Slightly upwards and horizontally toward the insertion as four muscular bands.
*Insertion:* Lower borders of last four ribs at the posterior side of the thoracic cage.
*Innervation:* Ventral rami of thoracic nerves.
*Function:* As Fig. 9 shows, the muscle can draw the lower ribs down during exhalation. The muscle can also act as a fixator for the lower four ribs preventing them being lifted as the diaphragma exerts pressure downwards on the abdominal viscera. Because many of the fibres course horizontally, the effect of pulling down on the ribs is probably only slight.

### d. Quadratus Lumborum

*General description:* Small, flat muscular sheet situated in the dorsal abdominal wall.
*Origin:* Top of iliac crest and the iliolumborum ligament which attaches to the transverse process of the fifth lumbar vertebra and the crest of the iliac.
*Course:* Upwards and somewhat medially.
*Insertion:* The last rib and upper four lumbar vertebrae.

*Innervation:* Lower thoracic and lumbar nerves.

*Function:* The main function of this muscle is probably to anchor the last rib (with the serratus posterior inferior) when the diaphragma contracts in inhalation. The muscle may also depress the last rib (see Fig. 9).

## B. Muscles of Inhalation (Those That Raise or Enlarge the Thoracic Cavity)

1. Thoracic Muscles

### a. Diaphragma (Diaphragm)

*General description:* Thin, but extremely strong, dome-shaped sheet of muscle separating the thoracic from the abdominal cavities.

*Origin:* A variety of attachments including the lower tip of the sternum, the first three or four lumbar vertebrae, the lower borders and inner surfaces of cartilages of ribs seven to twelve.

*Course:* The fibres course upwards and medially.

*Insertion:* All fibres insert into an irregularly shaped central tendon located nearer the front than the back. The muscle fibres and tendons comprise several intersecting layers which gives the diaphragma its great strength and special elastic properties.

*Innervation:* Phrenic nerve derived from the third, fourth and fifth cervical nerves.

*Function:* The main function of the muscle is to draw the central tendon down and slightly forward, thus enlarging the thoracic cavity in the vertical plane. Contraction of the diaphragma can also increase the antero-posterior and transverse dimensions of the thorax by elevating slightly the lower ribs. This effect of this activity, however, will be minimized if the ribs are fixed by the quadratus lumborum and serratus posterior inferior muscles.

The actual extent of movement of the diaphramga is probably only slight during normal speech. X-ray studies have shown a displacement of about 1–5 cm during normal and 10 cm during deep breathing (Wade, 1954). Nevertheless, many researchers (Hixon, 1973, p. 85) consider this displacement sufficient to account for most of the change in thoracic volume during normal inhalation. The electromyographic records of Ladefoged and his colleagues (Draper *et al.*, 1959, p. 20) show activity of the diaphragma all through inhalation and extending slightly into the exhalation phase.

When the diaphragma contracts, the increased pressure in the abdominal cavity causes the front abdominal wall to protrude. This action is illustrated schematically in Fig. 10. During exhalation the recoil

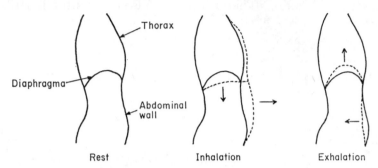

Fig. 10 A representation of the action of the diaphragma and the movement of the abdominal wall during inhalation and exhalation.

elasticity of the abdominal viscera displaces the diaphragma upwards and the abdominal wall returns to its initial shape.

### b. Intercostales Interni (Intercartilaginous Part)

The intercostales interni muscle has been discussed in Section II.A.1.a. Because of the particular shape of the intercartilaginous part of the muscle (i.e. the part between the costal cartilages near the sternum) many writers (Campbell, 1958; Zemlin, 1968, p. 91) have suggested that contraction of this part of the muscle can raise the ribs, thus having an inhalatory function. The function of the main part of the muscle is, however, exhalatory.

### c. Intercostales Externi (External Intercostals)

General description: Eleven pairs of thin muscles filling the intercostal spaces and lying just above the intercostales interni muscle. The muscle fibres are deficient near the sternum.
Origin: Lower border of each rib.
Course: Downwards and forwards, at right angles to the intercostales interni.
Insertion: Into the upper border of the rib below. In the lower spaces it merges with the obliquus externus muscle.
Innervation: Spinal intercostal nerves.
Function: When the first rib is fixed (e.g. by the scalenus muscles), the

intercostales externi can couple the ribs and raise the thoracic cage (see Fig. 11). Also, together with the intercostales interni, the muscle can help to strengthen the thoracic wall to prevent the intercostal spaces bulging in and out during breathing. Draper *et al.* (1959, p. 22)

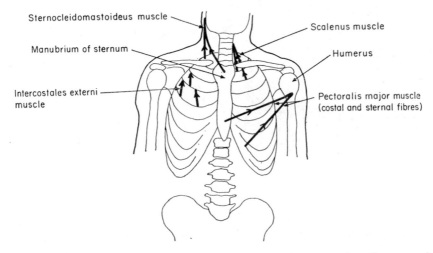

Fig. 11 Some directions of movement of the thoracic cage during contraction of some muscles of inhalation. (Intercostales externi muscles extend towards the sternum.)

have described a checking function of the muscle in preventing a too fast descent of the rib cage during exhalation.

## 2. Back Muscles (For Forced Inhalation)

### a. Serratus Posterior Superior

*General description:* Thin, wide muscle situated on the outer aspect of the ribs between the superficial and deep muscles of the back.
*Origin:* Last cervical and upper three or four thoracic vertebrae.
*Course:* Downward and laterally.
*Insertion:* Ribs two to five, lateral to the angles.
*Innervation:* First three or four thoracic nerves.
*Function:* Draws ribs upwards, acting mainly on their posterior sections (see Fig. 12).

### b. Latissimus Dorsi (Costal Fibres)

The latissimus dorsi has been discussed above in Section II.A.3.*a* as a muscle of exhalation. It was seen that when the arm is braced, contraction of the costal fibres can raise the lower three or four ribs,

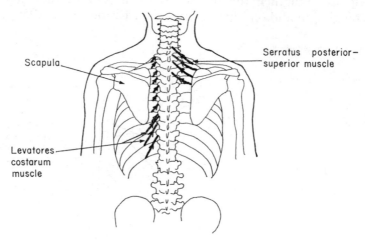

Fig. 12 The back view of the body showing some directions of movement of the thoracic cage during contraction of some muscles of inhalation.

although contraction of the muscle as a whole probably compresses the lower thoracic cage during exhalation.

### c. Levatores Costarum

*General description:* Twelve small slips of muscle located on the back of the thoracic cage.

*Origin:* Transverse process of the lowest cervical and upper eleven thoracic vertebrae.

*Course:* Downwards and somewhat laterally, diverging into fan-like ribbons which run almost parallel to the intercostales externi (see Fig. 12).

*Insertion:* Most fibres insert onto the back surfaces of the ribs immediately below the vertebrae of origin. The lowest fibres insert onto the second rib below.

*Innervation:* Spinal intercostal nerves.

*Function:* The main function of the muscle is probably to elevate the ribs but the fibres can also act to rotate, extend, or laterally flex the vertebral column. The muscle is sometimes regarded as a muscle of posture.

### d. Iliocostalis Cervicis

This muscle has been discussed above in Section II.A.3.b.

## 3. Neck Muscles

### a. Sternocleidomastoideus

*General description:* Strong, cylindrically-shaped, paired muscle situated along the sides of the neck.
*Origin:* Mastoid process of the temporal bone, just behind the ear.
*Course:* Downwards, dividing into two divisions—a sternal and a clavicular part.
*Insertion:* The sternal part inserts into the manubrium of the sternum, and the clavicular part into the top surface of the clavicle (see Fig. 11).
*Innervation:* Spinal root of accessory (eleventh cranial) nerve plus branches from cervical nerves two and three.
*Function:* The main function of the muscle is to rotate the head. However, with the head fixed, contraction of the muscle can probably raise the sternum and clavicle to increase the posterior–anterior dimension of the thorax during deep breathing.

### b. Scalenus

*General description:* The scalenus muscle consists of three groups of fibres situated on the side of the neck. The three groups are generally known as the scalenus anterior, the scalenus medius and the scalenus posterior.
*Origin:* The anterior arises from the third through sixth cervical vertebrae, the medius from the lower six cervical vertebrae, and the posterior from the lowest two or three cervical vertebrae.
*Course:* All fibres course vertically downwards.
*Insertion:* The anterior fibres insert into the upper surface of the first rib, the medius into the superior border of the first rib just behind the anterior, and the posterior into the outer surface of the second rib.
*Innervation:* Ventral rami of cervical nerves three to seven.
*Function:* The main function of the muscle is probably to raise the first and second ribs during inhalation (see Fig. 11). The muscle can also act as a fixator in bracing the upper ribs while the intercostales muscles contract. This bracing action can also help to prevent the thoracic cage being pulled down by the abdominal muscles.

## 4. Pectoral Muscles (For Forced Inhalation)

### a. Pectoralis Major

*General description:* Large, prominent, fan-shaped muscle situated on the superficial surface of the anterior wall of the thorax.
*Origin:* Greater tubercle of the humerus (the major bone of the upper arm).
*Course:* The fibres fan out widely as they travel across the thorax.
*Insertion:* A complex insertion including the medial half of the clavicle, the anterior surface of the sternum, and the second to the seventh costal cartilages.
*Innervation:* Medial and lateral anterior thoracic nerves from the brachial plexus.
*Function:* The primary function of the muscle is to act as an adductor of the arm. However, when the pectoral girdle is fixed, it may raise the ribs and sternum and so contribute to expansion of the thoracic cage (see Fig. 11).

### b. Pectoralis Minor

*General description:* Thin, triangular muscle found deep to the pectoralis major.
*Origin:* Front surface of the scapula.
*Course:* Downwards and medially.
*Insertion:* Second or third through fifth ribs near the costal cartilages.
*Innervation:* Medial anterior thoracic nerve.
*Function:* Main function is to lower the shoulder but if the pectoral girdle is fixed it may act synergistically with the pectoralis major in raising the upper ribs (see Fig. 13).

### c. Serratus Anterior

*General description:* Extremely powerful muscle of the shoulder girdle. It is quadrangular in shape and situated on the side of the thoracic cage.
*Origin:* Ventral aspect of vertebral border of the scapula.
*Course:* Downwards and forwards.
*Insertion:* The muscle inserts by means of several individual slips into the upper eight or nine ribs.
*Innervation:* Long thoracic nerve from the brachial plexus.
*Function:* When the scapula is fixed the muscle can raise the upper ribs thus contributing to inhalation. This activity probably only occurs during forced breathing.

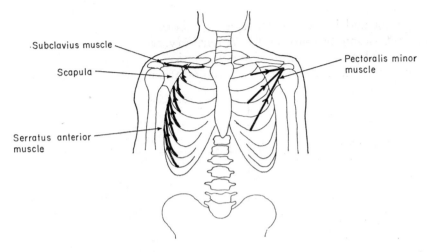

Fig. 13 Some directions of movement of the thoracic cage during contraction of some muscles of inhalation.

### d. Subclavius

*General description:* A small, cylindrically-shaped muscle situated on the underside of the clavicle.
*Origin:* Inferior surface of the clavicle.
*Course:* Medially and somewhat downward.
*Insertion:* Anterior surface of the junction of the first rib and its cartilage.
*Innervation:* Cervical nerves five and six from the lateral trunk of the brachial plexus.
*Function:* If the clavicle is braced, contraction can elevate the first rib. In view of the almost horizontal course of the muscle, however, this action is probably only slight (see Fig. 13).

## C. Sequence of Respiratory Muscular Activity

The various investigations carried out by Ladefoged (1967, pp. 1–50) and his associates have been concerned with the time course of respiratory muscular activity and how this activity relates to the mechanical properties of the respiratory system, and the demands placed on the system during speech production. The technique of electromyography was used to record the activity in six respiratory muscles, the diaphragma, intercostales externi, intercostales interni, rectus abdominis, obliquus externi abdominis, and latissimus dorsi, during an utterance after a deep breath. Figure 14 shows the sequence of muscular activity in the

six muscles. During deep inhalation before speech begins the diaphragma and intercostales externi are both active. As speech begins,
the relaxation pressure of the respiratory system is greater than the
sub-glottal pressure required by phonation. It appears that, for some
speakers at least, activity of the intercostales externi continues into the

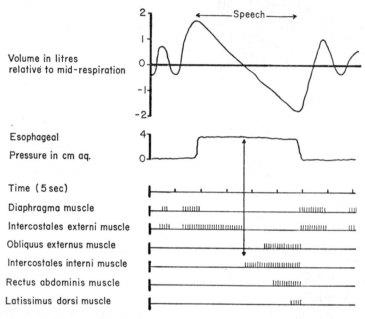

Fig. 14 The sequence of respiratory muscular activity during an utterance (counting from
1 to 32) spoken after a deep breath. The upper two graphs show records of the volume of air
in the lungs and the esophageal pressure respectively. (After Draper *er al.*, 1959.)

utterance thus serving to prolong this relaxation pressure. Then comes
(Draper *et al.*, 1960, p. 1843)

> "a short period when all muscles are inactive and the relaxation pressure
> acts alone; then expiratory muscles, beginning with the internal intercostals
> and later involving other muscles . . . reinforce the diminishing relaxation
> pressure."

The other accessory muscles are, for example, the rectus abdominis,
the obliquus externis abdominis and the latissimus dorsi. There is
reason to believe that other exhalatory muscles as well may be involved
in the regulation of respiratory pressures during speech.
   This sequence of muscular activity was produced during a long steady
utterance (counting) which can hardly be regarded as representative of

normal conversational speech. In conversational speech the demands placed on the respiratory system are quite different. Rapid fluctuations in pressure due to stop consonant occlusions, settings of the vocal folds, etc. occur extremely rapidly and must be compensated for by the respiratory system. According to Hixon (1973, p. 121), muscle spindle reflex systems associated with the intercostal muscles perform automatic length stabilization of the muscles to compensate for transient loading changes arising, for example, from supraglottal activity. The intercostal muscles are well suited to this task as their inherent characteristics allow them to contract extremely rapidly.


## III. Respiratory Activity Associated with Suprasegmental Features


It is now fairly well established that increased stress is associated with increased intensity arising from greater muscular tension being exerted in the respiratory system. Ladefoged (1967) in his electromyographic investigations, showed for some subjects an increase in activity of the intercostales interni preceding the principal stresses in an utterance. Other writers, e.g. Stetson (1951) have claimed stress involves the increased exhalatory activity of the abdominal musculature. It is probably true that some speakers use predominantly thoracic activity to expel air from the lungs, and others use abdominal activity. The reasons for the preference of one motion over the other is still uncertain; we need far more experimental data on sub-glottal pressures, lung volume displacements and electromyographic activity in the various respiratory muscles.

Increased activity in the respiratory muscles can alter not only the acoustic intensity of a sound but also its fundamental frequency ($f_0$). The relationship between sub-glottal pressure and $f_0$ is a little more complex, however, because of one's ability to alter $f_0$ at the level of the glottis itself, independently of any sub-glottal activity (MacNeilage, 1972, p. 7). The possible independence of $f_0$ and intensity changes is further illustrated by a language such as Serbo-Croatian where the correlation between intensity and $f_0$ changes can be rather low (Lehiste, 1970, p. 134). In English, however, stress is usually accompanied by an increase in both intensity and $f_0$ (Lehiste, 1970, pp. 106–153).

The relationship between respiratory activity and certain linguistic units such as the syllable has been investigated by Stetson (1951). He claimed that during speech production, abdominal muscles posture the thoracic cage while thoracic muscles, notably the intercostales interni, produce rapid breath pulse movements called chest pulses. These rapid ballistic-type pulses are said to be associated with production of syllables. Stetson's claims have since been refuted by Ladefoged (1967, p. 20) who found no easily identifiable peaks in intercostal activity associated with syllable production.

The relationship between respiratory activity and prosodic features such as $f_0$ and intensity will be touched on again in the next chapter where the physiology of laryngeal activity will be discussed.

# 4
# The Physiology of the Larynx

## I. General Description of the Larynx and its Associated Structure, the Hyoid Bone

In the previous chapter, it was seen how the respiratory system functions to produce a flow of air which passes out of the lungs and into the oral and nasal cavities (see Fig. 7). As the air passes out of the lungs and through these cavities it is modified by various structures, the first of which is the larynx. The primary biological function of the larynx is to act as a mechanical valve, if necessary closing off air from the lungs or preventing foreign substances (e.g. food) from entering the trachea. Apart from its important biological functions, however, the larynx is also necessary for speech production, in that it modifies the air-flow from the lungs in such a way as to produce an acoustic signal.

The larynx is generally regarded as consisting of nine cartilages: three unpaired (the thyroid, cricoid and epiglottis) and three paired (the arytenoid, corniculate and cuneiform cartilages). These cartilages are connected to each other by complex joints and move about these joints by means of various muscular and ligamentous forces. The motions of the various cartilages about these joints permit the wide variety of configurations that the larynx can assume during speech production.

Situated just above the larynx in the anterior part of the neck and intimately connected to it by muscles, is the horseshoe-shaped hyoid bone, which, incidentally, also serves as a base for the tongue. Because any movement of the hyoid bone potentially has an effect on the movement of the laryngeal cartilages, the physiology of the two structures will be discussed together in this chapter.

Before discussing in detail the muscular system of the larynx, it is useful to describe the major laryngeal cartilages and their movements about the various laryngeal joints.

## II. The Laryngeal Cartilages and Their Connecting Joints

The cricoid cartilage is a ring-shaped structure which is attached to the top of the trachea by means of a ligamentous connection. The esophagus,

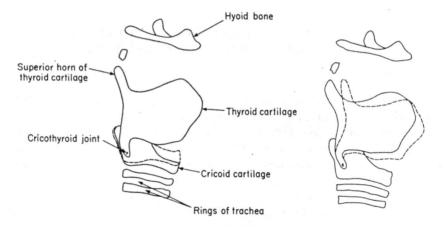

Fig. 15 Sagittal section illustrating the relationship between the cricoid cartilage, the thyroid cartilage and the hyoid bone, and two different viewpoints concerning the function of the cricothyroideus muscle. Left, an upward movement of the cricoid cartilage and right, a forward–downward tilting of the thyroid cartilage.

through which food passes into the stomach, lies immediately posterior to the cricoid. On the lower lateral surface of the cricoid are a pair of articular facets, to which the larger thyroid cartilage attaches, also by means of a ligament. The general shape of the thyroid and cricoid cartilages and two possible types of movement about the cricothyroid joint, is shown in Fig. 15. The figure shows how either the anterior part of the cricoid moves upwards, or the thyroid tilts forward, the extent of both movements being limited by the ligamentous connections. As will be shown later, the movement about this joint has an important function in the control of the frequency of vibration of the vocal cords.

Another important structure in the larynx is formed by the paired arytenoid cartilages, which are coupled by means of the cricoarytenoid joints to the posterior lateral part of the cricoid cartilage. These joints permit what is usually described as a rocking and gliding movement of the arytenoid cartilages (Sonesson, 1959; Von Leden and Moore, 1961) which is shown schematically in Fig. 16. The gliding movement enables the arytenoids to move parallel to the axes of the joints. The rocking movement is a rotation round the joints in a direction perpendicular to the axes of the joints. This motion can carry the arytenoid cartilages

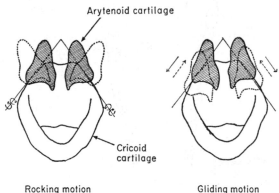

Rocking motion             Gliding motion

Fig. 16 The "rocking" and "gliding" motions of the arytenoid cartilages about the cricoary-tenoid joint (after Sonesson, 1970).

away from (abduction) or toward (adduction) the mid-sagittal plane. The vocal cords attach directly onto the arytenoid cartilages so any movement of these cartilages will have a direct influence on the configuration and tension of the cords. The cords themselves consist essentially of a pair of tough ligamentous membranes called the vocal ligaments, as well as a fibrous sheet called the conus elasticus, and muscle fibres. They form a slit-shaped opening, the glottis, which acts as a valve regulating the flow of air during speaking and breathing. A coronal cross-section through the larynx showing the relationship of the thyroid, cricoid and the glottis is shown in Fig. 17. The extent of the opening of the glottis is regulated mainly by movements of the arytenoid cartilages, a relatively adducted position being necessary for vibration to occur as in voiced sounds, and a relatively abducted position being necessary for normal breathing to occur.

The next cartilage, the epiglottis, is frequently described as a leaf-like structure, which attaches to the anterior part of the thyroid cartilage by means of a ligament. The upper free extremity lies just posterior to the back of the tongue, to which it attaches by means of membranous folds called the lateral and medial glossoepiglottic folds. The primary function of the epiglottis is to close off the entrance to the larynx during swallowing, to prevent food passing into the trachea. Two other sets of

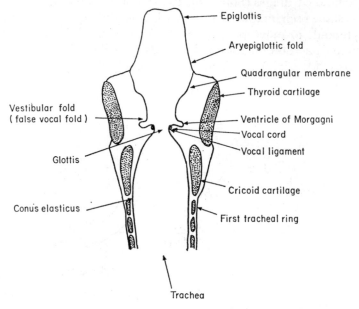

Fig. 17 A coronal section through the larynx showing some of its main structures.

cartilage, the so-called cuneiform cartilages of Wrisberg, and the corniculate cartilages of Santorini are of minor importnace and are not present in all larynges. The corniculate cartilages are small elastic cones which are attached to the apexes of the arytenoids. The cuneiform cartilages are in the form of narrow elongated rods which stretch from the sides of the epiglottis to the apexes of the arytenoid cartilages. When present, they probably lend support to the aryepiglottic folds at the entrance to the larynx vestibule.

## III. The Physiology of Laryngeal Movements

The muscles of the larynx can be divided up into an extrinsic and an intrinsic group. The extrinsic muscles are those which have their origins outside the larynx and attach onto various parts of the cartilaginous framework. They are probably mainly responsible for gross movements of the larynx as a whole and will only indirectly affect the vocal cords themselves. The intrinsic muscles, on the other hand, have both their origins and points of insertion within the larynx, and are directly responsible for modifying the configuration and tension of the vocal cords, by movement of the cricoid about the cricothyroid joint, by the rocking and gliding motion of the arytenoid cartilages, and by isometric contraction of muscles within the vocal cords themselves. The extrinsic group can be divided into those muscles which are situated above the hyoid bone—the so-called suprahyoid musculature, and those which are situated below the hyoid—the infrahyoid musculature.

The main laryngeal motions and configurations and the muscles primarily responsible for these actions are as follows:

## A. Extrinsic Muscles

1. Laryngeal elevators— suprahyoid group:
   - a. digastricus (anterior and posterior belly)
   - b. geniohyoideus
   - c. mylohyoideus
   - d. genioglossus
   - e. hyoglossus
   - f. stylohyoideus
   - g. constrictor pharyngis medius

2. Laryngeal depressors— infrahyoid group:
   - a. sternohyoideus
   - b. omohyoideus
   - c. thyrohyoideus
   - d. sternothyroideus

## B. Intrinsic Muscles

1. Sphincter muscles of laryngeal inlet:
   - a. aryepiglotticus
   - b. thyroepiglotticus
2. Abductor:
   - a. cricoarytenoideus posterior
3. Adductor:
   - a. cricoarytenoideus lateralis
   - b. arytenoideus transversus
   - c. arytenoideus obliquus
4. Tensor:
   - a. vocalis
   - b. cricothyroideus
5. Relaxer:
   - a. thyroarytenoideus externus

Figure 18 shows schematically the direction of movement of the hyoid bone and the laryngeal cartilages due to contraction of the ex-

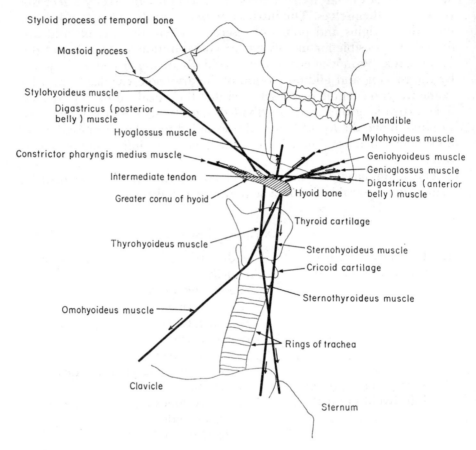

Fig. 18 The extrinsic laryngeal musculature showing the direction of movement of the hyoid bone, when the muscles contract from fixed origins.

trinsic laryngeal muscles. The figure clearly shows the great versatility of movement of the hyoid bone: a vertical upward–downward movement, as well as a forward–backward tilting movement, due to contraction of either the anterior or posterior suprahyoid muscles respectively.

Each muscle and its probable function will now be considered in more detail.

## A. Muscles Responsible for Gross Movements of the Larynx— the Extrinsic Laryngeal Muscles

### 1. Laryngeal Elevators (Suprahyoid Muscles)

#### a. Digastricus (Anterior and Posterior Belly

*General description:* The two bellies of the digastricus muscle, although functionally separate, are usually regarded as constituting the same muscle. Both bellies consist of long, thin muscle fibres, which connect in a common tendon near the hyoid bone (Fig. 18).

*Origin:* The anterior belly arises on the inner surface of the mandible close to the origin of the geniohyoideus (see below). The posterior belly arises in the mastoid process of the skull (Fig. 18).

*Course:* The anterior fibres course downwards and posteriorly; the posterior fibres, downwards and anteriorly.

*Insertion:* Both bellies insert in the intermediate tendon attached to the body of the hyoid bone, with fibres from both bellies interdigitating. a

*Innervation:* The anterior belly is served by the mylohyoideus nerve, derivative of the inferior alveolar branch of the trigeminal nerve. The posterior belly is supplied by the digastricus branch of the facial (seventh cranial) nerve.

*Function:* Due to their attachment to the hyoid bone, contraction of both bellies will tend to raise the hyoid and so the whole larynx to which it is attached. This elevation of the larynx is undoubtedly important in the second stage of swallowing to push the epiglottis up against the tongue and so help to prevent food entering the larynx. Raising of the larynx is also one way of decreasing the volume of the supra-glottal cavity and so increasing the supra-glottal pressure. Such activity may be necessary, for example, during the production of voiceless stops to prevent the occurrence of a sufficient trans-glottal pressure difference to cause vibration of the vocal cords. Vigorous raising of the larynx is undoubtedly important for creating a sufficiently high supra-glottal pressure during the production of ejectives such as [p'], [t'], [k'] (Ladefoged, 1973).

The posterior belly of the digastricus, because of the position of its origin, will tend to draw the hyoid bone upwards and posteriorly. This upward, posterior movement is probably important for bringing the back of the tongue (which attaches directly onto the hyoid) into position for the production of velar articulations such as [k], [u], etc. The anterior belly, on the other hand, when contracting from a fixed mandible, will act to bring the hyoid and so the tongue, anteriorly and upwards. Such a movement is important for alveolar articulations such as [t], [s], [i], where the whole body of the tongue is moved forward and upwards in the mouth. It is possible that the raising of the hyoid and so the larynx (particularly the thyroid cartilage), will tend to stretch and tense the vocal cords in the superior–inferior dimension, thus leading to a higher rate of vibration. This may be the reason for the frequently observed higher intrinsic pitch associated with close front and back vowels, such as [i], [u] (Lehiste, 1970, pp. 68–71).

### b. Geniohyoideus

*General description:* A short, cylindrical, paired muscle lying close to the mid-line of the floor of the mouth.

*Origin:* The muscle takes its origin from the anterior inner surface of the mandible, near the symphysis (Fig. 18).

*Course:* Downwards and posteriorly.

*Insertion:* The fibres insert into the anterior body of the hyoid bone.

*Innervation:* Loop between the first two cervical nerves.

*Function:* Together with the posterior fibres of the genioglossus, the anterior belly of the digastricus, and the mylohyoideus, the geniohyoideus helps to raise the hyoid upwards and forwards when the mandible is fixed (see Fig. 18). This action will raise both the tongue and the larynx (see above, under digastricus). The geniohyoideus may also act as antagonist to the thyrohyoideus (see below) in tilting the hyoid and so the thyroid cartilage backward. This action may be important for the production of velar and uvular articulations (Van Riper and Irwin, 1958, p. 366).

### c. Mylohyoideus

*General description:* The mylohyoideus consists of a thin sheet of fibres forming most of the muscular floor of the mouth. It lies just above the geniohyoideus.

*Origin:* The fibres arise from a groove called the mylohyoideus line running along the inner surface of the mandible back to a point almost adjacent to the second molar teeth.

*Course:* The fibres form a trough-like shape as they course downwards and medially.

*Insertion:* Fibres from both sides combine in a tendinous raphe which extends from the symphysis of the mandible to the hyoid bone.

*Innervation:* Mylohyoideus branch of the inferior alveolar nerve, part of the trigeminal (fifth cranial) nerve.

*Function:* The fibres act on the medial tendinous raphe to elevate the floor of the mouth and raise the hyoid bone forwards and upwards. In the latter movement the muscle acts in synergism with other elevators of the hyoid and larynx such as the geniohyoideus, digastricus, and genioglossus. Elevating the floor of the mouth is an important activity in swallowing.

Although the muscle is significant in bringing the tongue forward for articulations such as the alveolar consonants [l], [t], [n], it also plays a large part in bulging the tongue up and back for velar articulations (Hirano and Smith, 1967; Smith and Hirano, 1968). It probably acts here in synergism with suprahyoid muscles such as the posterior belly of the digastricus, stylohyoideus and constrictor pharyngis medius.

As with the other suprahyoid muscles, the mylohyoideus can be regarded as a muscle of the hyoid, the tongue, the mandible, or the larynx, depending on which of these structures is fixed by various fixator muscles, and what the function of the muscle is at any one time.

### d. Genioglossus

*General description:* The genioglossus is usually regarded as a muscle of the tongue because it constitutes most of the central muscular core of that organ (see Chapter 5). However, as the fibres attach to the hyoid bone, they can have some influence on raising the hyoid and larynx.
*Origin:* The muscle takes its origin from a tendinous connection fastened to the superior mental spine on the posterior border of the mandibular symphysis (Fig. 18).
*Course:* The anterior fibres curve fan-like in an anterior upward direction towards the tip of the tongue. The posterior fibres travel horizontally and backward towards the anterior surface of the hyoid bone and the interior surface of the base of the epiglottis. Most of the intermediate fibres travel in a medio-lateral direction. The course of the anterior and intermediate fibres is not shown in Fig. 18 but will be illustrated later in the description of muscles of the tongue.
*Insertion:* The anterior fibres insert in the tip of the tongue, there interdigitating with the inferior longitudinalis, the hypoglossus, and some fibres of the styloglossus (see Chapter 5, on muscles of the tongue). The intermediate fibres decussate with fibres from the opposite side, and with the superior longitudinalis and transversus tongue muscles.
*Innervation:* Hypoglossal (twelfth cranial) nerve.
*Function:* The posterior fibres can be regarded as elevators of the hyoid and larnyx when acting from a fixed mandible. In this action it assists the other anterior suprahyoid muscles such as *a.* (anterior belly), *b.* and

*c.* above. The function of the posterior and intermediate fibres in changing the position and configuration of the tongue will be discussed later in Chapter 5 under muscles of the tongue.

## *e. Hyoglossus*

*General description:* Like the genioglossus, the hyoglossus is usually regarded as a muscle of the tongue and will be described at greater length later in Chapter 5. It is a paired, quadrilateral sheet of muscle, lateral to the genioglossus.

*Origin:* Most of the fibres originate from the lateral part of the anterior surface of the body of the hyoid bone and also the whole extent of the greater cornu (see Fig. 18). The anterior fibres interdigitate at their origin with the superficial and deep fibres of the geniohyoideus.

*Course:* The most anterior fibres travel towards the tongue tip between the genioglossus medially and the mylohyoideus laterally. The posterior and middle fibres travel towards the root of the tongue.

*Insertion:* The anterior fibres attach to the mucous membrane of the tongue tip. Most of the posterior and medial fibres interdigitate with other tongue muscles such as the styloglossus and the lateral part of the inferior longitudinalis (see Chapter 5).

A small bundle of muscle fibres which originates from the lesser cornu of the hyoid bone courses parallel with the hyoglossus and inserts into the intrinsic muscles on the sides of the tongue. This bundle has been considered part of the hyoglossus muscle but some writers (Cunningham, 1972, p. 289) identify it as a separate muscle, the chondroglossus. The fibres, however, are not always present, so they are not treated as a separate muscle in this description.

*Innervation:* Hypoglossal (twelfth cranial) nerve.

*Function:* When the tongue is fixed by extrinsic tongue muscles such as the styloglossus and palatoglossus (see Chapter 5), contraction of the hyoglossus will tend to elevate the hyoid and so the larynx. The effect is similar to that achieved by the other suprahyoid muscles discussed above. The role of the hyoglossus in changing the position and configuration of the tongue will be discussed later in Chapter 5.

## *f. Stylohyoideus*

*General description:* Long, thin strip of muscle linking the hyoid bone to a fixed point on the skull.

*Origin:* The fibres arise from the styloid process on the temporal bone.

*Course:* Downward and anteriorly.

*Insertion:* Greater cornu of the hyoid bone (see Fig. 18)
*Innervation:* Stylohyoideus branch of facial (seventh cranial) nerve.
*Function:* The main function of this elevator of the hyoid bone is to work in synergism with the posterior belly of the digastricus in drawing the hyoid, and so the larynx, upwards and posteriorly. The posterior movement is probably aided by the constrictor pharyngis medius (see *g.* below) and may be important for velar and uvular articulations. Because the fibres attach to the greater cornu of the hyoid, any contraction will tend to tilt the hyoid and the thyroid cartilage forward, with the sternohyoideus (see Section III.A.2) acting as fixator (Fig. 18). This action may aid in bringing the tongue forward in the mouth for frontal articulations such as alveolar stops [t], [d] and inter-dental fricatives, e.g. [θ].

### g. Constrictor Pharyngis Medius

*General description:* This muscle is usually regarded as a muscle of the pharynx, being mainly responsible for contracting the pharynx during swallowing. Because, however, it attaches onto the hyoid bone it has some minor function as a larynx elevator.
*Origin:* Greater and lesser cornu of the hyoid.
*Course:* The fibres run fan-wise around the pharynx.
*Insertion:* The fibres insert into the posterior median raphe of the pharynx.
*Innervation:* The motor nerve supply is through the pharyngeal plexus into which passes the cranial root of the accessory (eleventh cranial) nerve.
*Function:* The muscle probably acts in synergism with the posterior belly of the digastricus and the stylohyoideus in moving the hyoid, and so the larynx as a whole, upwards and posteriorly. The effect of this muscle on the upward movement of the hyoid, however, is probably only slight, because of the almost horizontal course of the fibres.

## 2. Laryngeal Depressors (Infrahyoid Muscles)

### a. Sternohyoideus

*General description:* This muscle, which is usually described as one of the strap muscles of the neck is a long, flat, paired muscle.
*Origin:* The fibres arise from the posterior surface of the manubrium of the sternum and from the medial end of the clavicle.
*Course:* The muscle courses vertically, each side almost touching its fellow.

*Insertion:* Lower border of the body of the hyoid bone.

*Innervation:* Innervation is by the ansa cervicalis, the superior root of which runs with the hypoglossal.

*Function:* The main function of the muscle is to depress the hyoid and larynx when the sternum is fixed, thus acting antagonistically to the suprahyoid muscles. Lowering the larynx may serve a number of functions including lowering the fundamental frequency, by increasing the superior–inferior thickness of the vocal cords, and decreasing the supra-glottal pressure during the articulation of voiced lax stops such as [d], [g]. A vigorous lowering of the larynx takes place generally during the production of implosive stops which rely on a rapid decrease in supra-glottal and an increase in sub-glottal pressure.

Also, due to the muscle's insertion on the body of the hyoid bone, contraction will probably tilt down the anterior part of the hyoid. This tilting downward of the anterior part of the hyoid may occur during articulations made with the front part of the tongue.

The muscle can also theoretically act as an elevator of the sternum, and so the whole thoracic cage, when the hyoid is fixed by fixator muscles. This action, however, has yet to be supported experimentally.

### b. Omohyoideus

*General description:* Long narrow muscle, consisting of two bellies, a superior and an inferior, situated on the antero-lateral surface of the neck.

*Origin:* The inferior belly arises from the upper border of the scapula.

*Course:* The inferior belly passes anteriorly and upwards to insert into an intermediate tendon just beneath the sternocleidomastoideus muscle (one of the muscles of the neck). From this tendon, the superior belly courses vertically upwards (see Fig. 18).

*Insertion:* The superior belly inserts into the lower border of the hyoid bone.

*Innervation:* Same as sternohyoideus.

*Function:* The function of this muscle in lowering the hyoid and larynx is similar to that of the sternohyoideus discussed above.

### c. Thyrohyoideus

*General description:* A broad, thin muscle situated on the anterolateral surface of the neck.

*Origin:* Oblique line of the thyroid cartilage, passing over the thyrohyoid membrane.

*Course:* Vertically upwards.

*Insertion:* Lower border of the body and adjacent parts of the greater cornu of the hyoid (Fig. 18).

*Innervation:* The innervation of this muscle comes from a loop between the first and second cervical nerves.

*Function:* The thyrohyoideus can act in synergism with other infrahyoid muscles in depressing the hyoid and possibly also the thyroid cartilage. With the hyoid fixed, however, the muscle can raise the thyroid which may be important for example in producing a higher fundamental frequency (see discussion of suprahyoid muscles above).

Because of its insertion in the greater cornu of the hyoid, any contraction of the thyrohyoideus will tend to tilt the hyoid backwards. This may produce an appropriate position of the hyoid for the production of velar and uvular articulations.

### d. Sternothyroideus

*General description:* Long, thin muscle located in the anterior part of the neck beneath the omohyoideus and sternohyoideus muscles.

*Origin:* Posterior surface of the manubrium of the sternum and the first costal cartilage.

*Course:* The fibres course vertically upward and somewhat laterally.

*Insertion:* The fibres insert along the oblique line of the outer part of the thyroid cartilage.

*Innervation:* Ansa cervicalis.

*Function:* The sternothyroideus probably acts in synergism with the other infrahyoid muscles in lowering the larynx. It is possible that the muscle will cause some rotation in the cricothyroid joint. This movement would probably cause a shortening of the vocal cords, thus resulting in a lowered rate of vibration.

## B. Muscles Responsible for Changes in the Internal Configuration of the Larynx and the Vocal Cords—the Intrinsic Laryngeal Muscles

### 1. Sphincter Muscles of the Laryngeal Inlet

#### a. Aryepiglotticus

*General description:* The muscle is regarded by some as part of the superior fibres of the arytenoideus obliquus muscle situated along the lateral sides of the epiglottis.

*Origin:* Lateral part and apex of the arytenoid cartilage.
*Course:* Upwards and forwards.
*Insertion:* Lateral edges of epiglottis and quadrangular membrane (see Fig. 17).
*Innervation:* Inferior recurrent branch of the vagus (tenth cranial) nerve.
*Function:* This muscle serves primarily a protective function in closing off the entrance to the laryngeal vestibule by a sphincter action. This activity may occur for example during swallowing, so preventing food passing into the larynx. The muscle acts primarily in synergism to the arytenoideus obliquus muscle (see below).

### b. *Thyroepiglotticus*

*General description:* The muscle is thin and variable, exerting its main influence on the aryepiglottic folds and the epiglottis (see Fig. 17).
*Origin:* Inner surface of thyroid cartilage close to its angle.
*Course:* Upwards and posteriorly just above the thyroarytenoideus muscle.
*Insertion:* Aryepiglottic fold and the margin of the epiglottis.
*Function:* The muscle can act to depress the epiglottis thus closing off the laryngeal vestibule. The role of this muscle in speech production is uncertain at present.

## 2. Abductor Muscle

### a. *Cricoarytenoideus Posterior*

*General description:* The muscle acts to rotate the arytenoid cartilages outwards and is thus regarded as an abductor of the vocal cords. It is a broad, fan-shaped muscle.
*Origin:* The fibres arise from a depression on the posterior surface of the cricoid cartilage.
*Course:* Upwards and laterally with both sides converging.
*Insertion:* The posterior surface of the muscular process of each arytenoid.
*Innervation:* Inferior recurrent branch of the vagus (tenth cranial) nerve.
*Function:* The main function of the muscle is to pull the muscular process of the arytenoids diagonally downwards and towards the mid-line, thus rotating them on the cricoarytenoid joints. This results in the abduction of the cartilages and the consequent widening of the glottis (Fig. 19 illustrates this schematically). At the same time, because of the

position and nature of the cricoarytenoid joints, the vocal processes are projected slightly upwards. Electromyographic investigations by Hirose and Gay (1972, p. 158) have illustrated increased activity in this muscle in the production of voiceless stops and fricatives in both medial

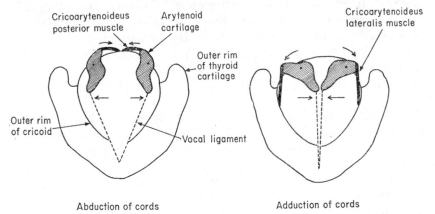

Abduction of cords                    Adduction of cords

Fig. 19 View of the glottis from above showing the abduction and adduction actions of the cricoarytenoideus posterior and the cricoarytenoideus lateralis respectively.

and final position. The activity was found to decrease for vowel production.

The muscle probably does not contract in an all-or-none fashion but is finely controlled by simultaneous activity of antagonist muscles such as the arytenoideus transversus, one of the main adductors of the cords.

## 3. Adductor Muscles

### a. Cricoarytenoideus Lateralis

*General description:* A small, quadrilateral-shaped muscle on the lateral wall of the larynx deep to the thyroid cartilage. The medial surface of the muscle is in contact with the conus elasticus.

*Origin:* The upper border of the arch of the cricoid cartilage.

*Course:* The fibres travel upwards and posteriorly along the rim of the cricoid.

*Insertion:* The fibres converge to insert on the muscular process in the lateral part of the arytenoid cartilage (Fig. 19).

*Innervation:* Inferior recurrent branch of the vagus (tenth cranial) nerve.

*Function:* The main function of the muscle is to rotate the arytenoids in their rocking motion, thus drawing the vocal processes together during the production of voiced articulations (Fig. 19). In approximating the vocal cords, the muscle acts as one of the main antagonist muscles to the cricoarytenoideus posterior, and a synergist to the arytenoideus transversus (see below). When the arytenoid cartilages are adducted for phonation, additional isotonic tension in the cricoarytenoideus lateralis will probably cause an increase in medial compression of the vocal cords, thus leading to a higher rate of vibration of the cords. In regulating fundamental frequency the muscle presumably acts in synergism with the cricothyroideus, and the vocalis muscles (Hirano et al., 1969, p. 624).

It is possible also that the cricoarytenoideus lateralis has a compensatory function, keeping the vocal cords together in a position appropriate for voicing during forceful contraction of the cricothyroideus for high pitches. This action may be necessary because forceful contraction of the cricothyroideus will tend not only to elongate the cords but also to abduct them slightly. According to Zemlin (1968, p. 152) the cricoarytenoideus lateralis can shape the glottis for the production of whisper. In this action the tips of the arytenoids are approximated and, upon further contraction of the muscle, the bodies are forced apart creating a wedge-shaped orifice through which the airstream passes.

### b. Arytenoideus Transversus

*General description:* The muscle is a thick, rectangular mass covering the entire posterior surface of the arytenoids. It is an unpaired muscle.
*Origin:* Posterior surface and lateral border of one arytenoid.
*Course:* Horizontal.
*Insertion:* Lateral edge and muscular process of the other arytenoid.
*Innervation:* Inferior recurrent branch of the vagus (tenth cranial) nerve.
*Function:* The muscle draws the arytenoids together mainly by their gliding motion but also partly by the rocking action about the cricoarytenoid joints (Fig. 20). Both activities draw the vocal cords together so allowing vibration to occur during voiced articulations. In addition to this basic activity in approximating the vocal cords for phonation, the muscle can probably exert some medial compression on the cords thus raising the fundamental frequency.

### c. Arytenoideus Obliquus

*General description:* A paired muscle placed externally on the arytenoideus transversus muscle.

*Origin:* Lower posterior surface of one arytenoid.
*Course:* Upwards and obliquely, the two sets of fibres crossing over each other. This gives the muscle a characteristic X shape when viewed from behind.
*Insertion:* Apex and lateral sides of the adjacent arytenoid, some fibres joining the aryepiglotticus muscle.
*Innervation:* Inferior recurrent branch of the vagus (tenth cranial) nerve.
*Function:* The muscle adducts the vocal cords by bringing the apexes

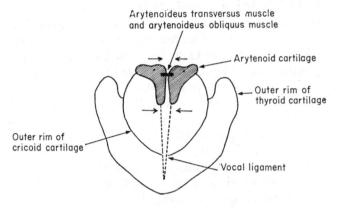

Adduction of cords

Fig. 20 The glottis showing the adduction effect of the arytenoideus transversus and the arytenoideus obliquus muscles.

of the arytenoid cartilages together thus acting synergistically to the arytenoideus transversus. During forced contraction the muscle can bring the vestibular folds closer together (Van Riper and Irwin, 1958, p. 434) resulting in a partial closure of the air-way. The type of voice quality this forced contraction causes is generally known as ventricular voice.

Contraction of this muscle, together with the aryepiglotticus will result in closing the vestibule of the larynx. This sphincter action, as mentioned above, mainly serves a protective function.

## 4. Tensor Muscles

### a. Vocalis

*General description:* With some fibres of the thyroarytenoideus externus muscle, the vocalis constitutes the muscular part of the vocal cords themselves.

*Origin:* Posterior lower half of the angle of the thyroid cartilage.

*Course:* Most fibres course in a posterior direction, diverging slightly.

*Insertion:* The uppermost fibres insert into the vocal processes of the arytenoid cartilages near the vocal ligament. Other fibres probably insert directly into the vocal ligament itself but this has not yet been definitely established.

*Innervation:* Inferior recurrent branch of the vagus (tenth cranial) nerve.

*Function:* The vocalis muscle is often regarded as an internal vocal cord tensor which functions mainly to achieve fine isometric tension in the cords. Isometric tension such as this would tend to stiffen the cords and so raise the pitch of the voice. According to some recent electromyographic research (Hirose and Gay, 1972, p. 160) the vocalis muscle is particularly active in voicing, being capable of rapid changes in tension, so providing fine adjustments to the cords.

Another possible function of the vocalis muscle is to actively shorten the vocal cords thus slackening the tension in the cords and so decreasing the fundamental frequency of phonation. In this isotonic activity, the vocalis would be acting antagonistically to muscles which lengthen the cords such as the cricothyroideus (see Section II.2.4.*b*).

The inherent characteristics of the vocalis muscle give clues as to its possible importance for speech production. According to a number of researchers (Fink, 1962; Broad, 1973; Lullies, 1977, p. 223,) the muscle has a particularly rich innervation with probable extremely low innervation ratios in the motor units. This would enable the CNS to exert very precise control over the contractual activity in the muscle—a factor which would be important for instance in achieving finely graded configurations necessary for different aspects of phonation such as the control of voice quality etc. The actual diverse arrangement of the muscular fibres also, with some fibres coursing parallel to the vocal ligaments and others perhaps inserting into the ligaments themselves would permit a great variety of movement.

At present, however, we can only speculate as to the precise function of this muscle. Instrumental techniques such as electromyography will hopefully provide more clues as to the function of this muscle during speech production.

### b. Cricothyroideus

*General description:* A broad, paired muscle superficially placed upon the larynx and divided into two muscular groups—the pars recta and the pars obliqua. The muscle is generally regarded as the main laryngeal regulator of pitch.

*Origin:* Both groups of fibres arise from the lower border and outer surface of the cricoid arch.

*Course:* The pars recta group of fibres course vertically upwards, while the pars obliqua course upwards and posteriorly.

*Insertion:* The pars recta fibres insert along the inner aspect of the lower margin of the thyroid cartilage, the pars obliqua insert into the anterior margin of the inferior cornu of the thyroid.

*Innervation:* Superior recurrent branch of the vagus (tenth cranial) nerve.

*Function:* The muscle functions primarily to rotate the cricoid cartilage

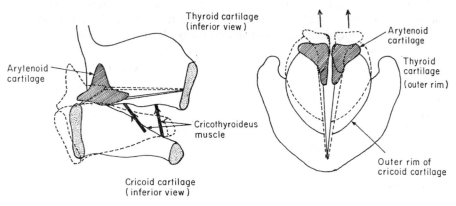

Fig. 21 The action of the cricothyroideus muscle in rotating the cricoid cartilage about the cricothyroid joint (left) and so elongating the vocal cords (right).

about the cricothyroid joint (see above). Because of the position of this joint, contraction of the cricothyroideus can raise the anterior part of the cricoid towards the anterior part of the thyroid, at the same time tilting the posterior part of the cricoid backwards. This activity will increase the distance between the angle of the thyroid cartilage and the arytenoids so extending, by a proportional amount, the length of the vocal cords (Fig. 21). This stretching, elongating action on the vocal cords will cause them to snap back more rapidly when air is passed through them during speech production, so increasing their rate of vibration. A number of recent electromyographic studies (Faaborg-Anderson, 1965; Shipp and McGlone, 1971; Sawashima, 1974; Sawashima *et al.*, 1969) have shown a positive correlation between increased activity in this muscle and increase in fundamental frequency.

Another possible function of this muscle is to tilt the thyroid cartilage forwards and downwards when acting from a fixed cricoid (Zemlin, 1968, p. 155; Sawashima, 1974). This tilting downward will have much the same function in elongating and tensing the vocal cords as rotation of the cricoid. In tensing the vocal cords, the muscle probably acts synergistically with the vocalis and thyroarytenoideus externus. Indeed, activity in both these muscles has been observed during increased fundamental frequency of phonation (Shipp *et al.*, 1972). The activity of the cricothyroideus in stretching and tensing the vocal cords could also be viewed as an antagonist activity to that of extrinsic laryngeal muscles such as the sternothyroideus which lower the thyroid cartilage so slackening the tension on the vocal cords in a vertical dimension. Recent studies (Harris, 1974) have suggested, however, that lowering of fundamental frequency may be a passive movement, simply a cessation of activity in the cricothyroideus and other muscles such as the vocalis and thyroarytenoideus externus which normally increase the tension in the vocal cords.

Forceful contraction of the cricothyroideus may cause a slight abduction of the cords. This is likely to occur for example at very high pitches. In order to maintain voicing by approximating the cords, antagonist activity by the vocal cord adductor muscles such as the cricoarytenoideus lateralis, the arytenoideus transversus, and the arytenoideus obliquus probably takes place.

## 5. Relaxer Muscle

### a. Thyroarytenoideus Externus

*General description:* The thyroarytenoideus externus muscle together with the vocalis muscle (which incidentally is sometimes regarded as a medially placed subdivision of the larger thyroarytenoideus muscle) make up the muscles within the vocal cords. Some researches (MacNeilage, 1972, p. 13) doubt whether there is any functional difference between the vocalis and the thyroarytenoideus externus muscle.
*Origin:* Inner surface of the thyroid cartilage at the angle.
*Course:* Posteriorly, in general parallel to the vocal ligament and most of the fibres of the vocalis muscle.
*Insertion:* Most of the fibres insert over a fairly large area of the anterolateral surface of the arytenoid cartilage. Some fibres continue round the lateral border of the arytenoid to interdigitate with the arytenoideus obliquus muscle. Other fibres interdigitate with the cricoarytenoideus lateralis.
*Innervation:* Inferior recurrent branch of vagus (tenth cranial) nerve.
*Function:* The main function of the muscle is probably to draw forward the arytenoid cartilages, thus shortening and relaxing the vocal cords.

In this activity the muscle would be antagonist to the cricothyroideus which stretches the cords.

Another possible function of the muscle would be to increase the isometric tension in the cords thus assisting the vocalis muscle. This latter activity could occur for example during increases in fundamental frequency. It is not yet firmly established just what the primary function of this muscle is in regulating fundamental frequency. It is possible that, like the vocalis muscle, its functions are primarily to determine the delicate configurations and different tension in the cords appropriate for various aspects of speech production.

Van Riper and Irwin (1958, p. 435) hypothesize that, if the cricothyroideus and cricoarytenoideus lateralis remain constant and the thyroarytenoideus relaxes, this will lead to a lowering of pitch and an increase in loudness. The increase in loudness would occur because the vocal cords are blown further apart with the same amount of air pressure when they are relaxed than when they are tensed. Hirose and Gay (1972) have found higher electromyographic activity for this muscle during the production of stressed vowels.

It is therefore possible to view this muscle either as a relaxer of the vocal cords or as a tensor, the former activity leading to a decrease in fundamental frequency and the latter to an increase.

## IV. The Laryngeal Control of Voicing, Pitch and Intensity

During voicing, the vocal cords are set in vibration by a complex combination of aerodynamic, muscular and elastic forces in the larynx. According to the generally accepted aerodynamic–myoelastic theory of voice production (Van den Berg, 1958), the first stage of the phonation process involves the build-up of air pressure below the vocal cords, which are approximated by the adductor muscles. When the sub-glottal pressure becomes great enough to overcome the resistance offered by the approximated cords they will be forced apart and air will flow through the glottal opening. As the air flows through the narrow glottis, the velocity will increase thus causing a decrease in intra-glottal pressure. (This fact is governed by Bernoulli's law, a discussion of which can be found in Broad, 1973, p. 141 *et seq.*) The decrease in pressure, plus the effect of the elastic forces in the tissue of the vocal cords themselves, will literally suck the cords medially together again. When the sub-glottal air pressure increases again sufficiently to force the

84 PHYSIOLOGY OF SPEECH PRODUCTION

cords apart, the cycle will be repeated. The resulting pulsing of air through the glottis generates a sound source, the frequency of which is determined by the rate of pulses, and the intensity by the sound pressure wave produced.

In actual fact the glottal wave form is extremely complex, mainly because different parts of the vocal cords vibrate in different ways. For example, at the start of the opening phase, under the influence of the increasing air pressure from the lungs, the most compliant area of the cords will begin to vibrate first. The deflection will shift to less compliant areas until the complete vocal cords are forced apart. Also, during the opening phase, the cords themselves are usually blown slightly upwards.

The picture is further complicated by the fact that the vocal cords need not necessarily be completely closed in the prephonatory stage for vibration to occur. In the production of so-called breathy voice, for example, vibration occurs without the vocal cords actually closing. This will produce a certain amount of turbulent noise simultaneous with voicing.

In Korean this occurs at the beginning of vibration for a vowel following the release for a tense aspirated stop (Hardcastle, 1973). During the production of the stop the vocal cords are held fairly far apart (Kim, 1970; Fujimura, 1972, p. 133; Kagaya, 1971) and this abducted position continues into the first few cycles of the vowel. Vibration occurs because the air-flow is relatively high, and the muscles in the vocal cords are under increased isometric tension. This slightly abducted position of the cords will usually cause a certain amount of turbulent noise to occur, which can easily be seen in the acoustic wave-form (Hardcastle, 1973).

Many factors other than aerodynamic forces will influence the nature of the vocal cord vibration. The elastic and muscular forces in the larynx, for example, can determine the speed at which the vocal cords snap back into place during the vibratory cycle. Also, the configuration and tension of the vocal cords themselves can determine a large range of different voice qualities, for example, "creaky voice" where the vocal cords are considerably thickened and vibrate only in the anterior part at a very low frequency (McGlone and Shipp, 1971, p. 774), and "falsetto voice" where the vocal cords are so elongated and tensed that only the medial edges vibrate (Judson and Weaver, 1965, p. 73). A complete physiological description of different voice qualities has not yet been carried out. Such a description would be extremely valuable in speech therapy where different voice qualities may be important indications of certain pathological conditions in the larynx.

ⅴ The frequency at which the vocal cords vibrate determines the pitch of the voice and depends on a number of factors, the most important of which are A. the longitudinal length of the cords, B. the muscular tension within the cords, C. the rate of the air-flow through the glottis (which depends in part on the sub-glottal pressure), D. medial compression on the cords, and E. the height of the larynx.

## A. Longitudinal Length

Many investigations (Arnold, 1961; Hollien and Moore, 1960; Sonesson, 1970) have found a direct correlation between the fundamental frequency ($f_0$) of phonation and the longitudinal length of the vocal cords; as the length increases, $f_0$ is raised. The increase in length is mainly accomplished by the combined action of the cricothyroideus muscle which causes rotation about the cricothyroid joint, and the cricoarytenoideus lateralis, which prevents abduction of the cords during the rotary movement. Electromyographic activity has been registered in both these muscles during increases in $f_0$ (Hirano et al., 1969). As the cords are elongated they will become tauter and thinner. The vibrating mass will thus become less and the cords will be both easier to move and will accelerate more rapidly during the phonatory cycle. Numerous laminagraphic studies (Hollien, 1962; Hollien and Coltan, 1969), have demonstrated that decrease in vocal cord mass (thickness) is closely correlated with $f_0$ change in the normal frequency range.

## B. Muscular Tension

Another factor which influences the frequency of vibration of the cords is the change in tension in the vocalis and thyroarytenoideus muscles in the cords themselves. When the tension is isotonic, the cords will be shortened, thus opposing the activity of the cricothyroideus. The shorter, thicker cords will then presumably vibrate slower. If, however, the muscles are tensed isometrically there will be no shortening and the muscles will become tauter and stiffer. This will probably have the same effect as the cricothyroideus in raising the $f_0$.

## C. Rate of Air-flow and/or Sub-glottal Pressure Differences

The rate of air-flow through the glottis depends partly on the sub-glottal pressure and will largely determine the degree to which the

Bernoulli effect sucks the cords towards each other. However, it is not entirely clear at present just what the relative contributions of adjustments at the larynx and sub-glottal air pressure are to changes in $f_0$ (MacNeilage, 1972). It seems from recent research (Hixon *et al.*, 1970) that variance in $f_0$ cannot be accounted for solely in terms of sub-glottal pressure differences.

One factor which probably influences the variation in $f_0$ is the degree of tension within the cords themselves. When the cords are under isometric tension a greater sub-glottal pressure is required to force them apart than when they are relaxed and loose. The greater sub-glottal pressure will cause an increased rate of air-flow through the glottis, thus tending to raise the $f_0$ and also the intensity of the resulting phonation.

At normal pitch ranges it is probable, therefore, that both air-flow and laryngeal tension contribute to changes in $f_0$. At high pitches, however, because the vocal cords are already under almost maximum tension due to cricothyroideus, vocalis and thyroarytenoideus activity, $f_0$ is probably controlled mainly by rate of air-flow through the glottis (Isshiki, 1969).

## D. Medial Compression

Another force in the larynx which can also regulate $f_0$ is the degree of medial compression on the vocal cords exerted by the arytenoid cartilages. As we saw above in the discussion of the laryngeal adductor muscles (the cricoarytenoideus lateralis, the arytenoideus transversus, and the arytenoideus obliquus), contraction of these muscles can press the vocal processes of the arytenoids together for vibration to occur. If the activity is increased, a medial force on the posterior part of the vocal cords could be imposed thus leaving only the anterior part free to vibrate (Van den Berg and Tan, 1959; Broad, 1973, p. 152). If vibration does occur under these conditions it is usually at a higher rate because the mass of the cords available for vibration is decreased.

## E. Height of the Larynx

As we mentioned above in the description of the extrinsic laryngeal muscles, activity in these muscles could theoretically alter the $f_0$ by raising or lowering the laryngeal cartilages (particularly the thyroid) thus increasing or decreasing the tension of the cords in their superior–

inferior plane. One would expect then increased activity in the laryngeal elevators such as the geniohyoideus, digastricus, genioglossus, mylohyoideus, etc. at higher $f_0$, and increase in the laryngeal depressors such as sternohyoideus, sternothyroideus and omohyoideus at lower $f_0$. This hypothesis, however, is yet to be conclusively tested by electromyographic techniques.

It is clear from the above discussion that increased air-flow through the glottis leading to higher sound intensity is almost invariably accompanied by an increase in $f_0$. This physiological observation has important phonetic implications particularly as regards the acoustic correlates of prosodic features such as intonation and stress patterns. Two of the most commonly observed correlates of increased stress in English are increased intensity (with associated increase in sub-glottal pressure and air-flow) and increased $f_0$ (Lieberman, 1960; Jassem and Morton, 1965; Ladefoged, 1967; Lehiste, 1970, Ch. 4).

The next chapter will discuss the physiology of articulatory movements within the vocal tract, where the sound wave generated at the glottis is modified to produce intelligible speech.

# 5

# The Physiology of Articulatory Organs in the Vocal Tract

## I. General Outline of the Vocal Tract

In the previous chapter, we discussed the various ways in which the vocal cords can function to modify the flow of air generated by the respiratory system: they can be completely closed (glottal stop) shutting off the flow of air; they can be approximated to enable vibration to occur, or they can be abducted to allow the air to flow relatively unimpeded through. The articulatory organs in the vocal tract above the glottis have the important function of either modifying the sound source produced at the glottis (which happens for example during the production of voiced sounds), or interrupting the air-flow by complete or partial constriction somewhere in the vocal tract. Complete obstruction of the air-flow occurs, for example, during the occlusion phase of stop production, and partial constriction occurs during fricative production, where turbulent noise is generated at the point of constriction. In this chapter the various articulatory organs that fulfil these functions will be described.

Figure 22 shows a schematic diagram of the most important articulators and their associated structures in the oral and nasal cavities. The most important articulators are the soft palate or velum, the tongue, pharynx, lips and mandible. An important associated structure is the hard palate, which forms part of the skeletal framework of the skull, and contains the upper teeth and gums. All of the articulators except the pharynx, and to a lesser extent the soft palate, are very mobile structures, being capable of relatively fast movements and a wide range of different

configurations. The inherent speed and versatility of movement, however, differs among the articulators themselves. The tongue, for
example, is by far the most mobile structure achieving an almost in-
finite variety of postures and configurations. According to research by
Hudgins and Stetson (1937, p. 92), the tongue tip is capable of the

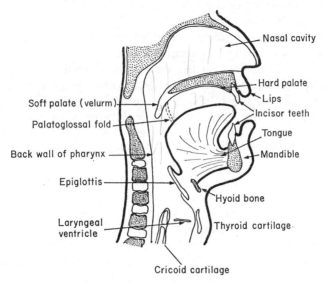

Fig. 22 The oral and nasal cavities showing the relative positions of the various articulatory
organs.

fastest movements of all the articulators (from 7·2–9·6 movements per
sec). Rates of movement for the other articulators were given as:

| | |
|---|---|
| Mandible | 5·9–8·4(movements per sec) |
| Back part of tongue | 5·4–8·9 |
| Velum | 5·2–7·8 |
| Lips | 5·7–7·7 |

The same progression for the mandible, tongue, and lips was found by
Kaiser (1934, p. 123). Kaiser, however, found also that some lip movement parameters could be executed more rapidly than others. For
example, the lowering and raising of the lower lip could be produced more
rapidly than its protrusion and retraction. It was also suggested that
lowering the mandible occurred faster than raising it.
    Most of these differences in the speed of movement of the various
articulators can be explained with reference to the inherent properties
of the muscular systems associated with movement of the articulators,

and the mechanical constraints imposed on the movement by differences in mass, inertia, force of gravity etc. One criterion is the size and type of muscles used in moving the articulator (see Chapter 2). For example, the small, intrinsic muscles of the tongue, which are responsible for moving the tip, are capable of extremely fast, precisely controlled activity. The lowering of the jaw also is performed by activity of short, powerful, rapidly contracting muscles such as the anterior part of the genioglossus, the geniohyoideus, and anterior belly of the digastricus, with gravity also playing a synergistic role.

Movements of the lips, on the other hand, particularly the closing and rounding–protruding movements, involve primarily the slower, sphincter activity of the relatively large orbicularis oris muscle. Such intrinsic constraints on the physiological activity of the articulators undoubtedly play an important role in the serial ordering and motor control of speech production. It is probable that accurate specifications of the intrinsic properties of the articulatory organs are stored in the brain as part of the motor *schema* for various articulatory movements.

Figure 22 illustrates the intricate interdependence of the articulators during speech production. It can be seen, for example, how movements of the tongue can alter both the width of the pharynx and the height of the larynx; how movements of the mandible can affect the configuration and posture of the lower lip, as well as the position and, to a lesser extent, the shape of the tongue; and how movements of the velum can alter the shape of the back part of the tongue, because of muscular connections between the two articulators.

The remainder of this chapter will be devoted to a more detailed discussion of the physiology of each articulatory organ and its probable role in speech production, beginning with the most important articulator, the tongue.

## II. Physiology of Lingual Movements

### A. General Outline of the Structure of the Tongue

As is shown in Fig. 22 the tongue is shaped a little like an inverted shoemaker's iron with the inferior part attached to the hyoid bone. The substance of the tongue is mainly muscle with a mucous membrane covering (called the epithelium), a lamina propria of connective tissue, glands and lymph nodules (Cunningham, 1972, p. 409). Anatomically, the organ can be divided into two parts—the oral and pharyngeal, usually separated by a V-shaped furrow on the upper surface of the dorsum (see Fig. 23). The oral part comprises two-thirds of the body of the tongue and is that part which is freely moveable in the mouth. It is loosely attached to the floor of the mouth by a membranous fold called the frenulum, which is visible when the tongue tip is raised and retracted. The more fixed, pharyngeal part of the tongue is anchored securely

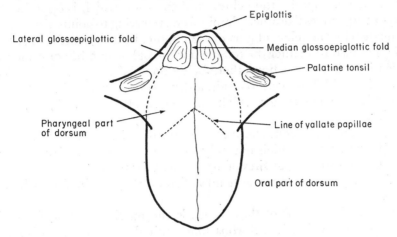

Fig. 23 The tongue dorsum and the top edge of the epiglottis showing the glossoepiglottic folds.

by muscle to the hyoid bone, and to the styloid process of the skull. It lies just anterior to the epiglottis, which is connected to it by the median glossoepiglottic and the two lateral glossoepiglottic folds (Fig. 23).

The dorsum or upper surface of the tongue is coated with small punctiform projections called papillae each containing a core of connective tissue and covered by the epithelium. Four types of lingual papillae have been identified on the anterior aspect of the tongue: filiform, fungiform, vallate and foliate papillae (Sognnaes, 1954). Within each of these papillae some form of nerve ending has been found (Dixon, 1962), the fungiform and vallate being particularly well endowed with taste buds. Immediately below the papillae projections is fatty tissue containing blood vessels, serous glands and nerve fibres. Because of the complex interlacing of nerve fibres in the connective tissue and subpapillary region, it is extremely difficult to isolate individual nerve endings. A good review of the histological work relating to sensory endings in the papillary and sub-papillary tissues can be found in Grossman and Hattis (1967).

Phoneticians have divided the dorsum into a number of divisions on a hypothecated functional basis. Pike (1943, p. 120), for example, has

"convenient arbitrary points of reference"

which he calls the tip or apex, the blade, and middle (cf. Gimson, 1970, p. 8), which are those parts directly beneath the hard palate, the back, which is opposite the velum, and the root, which is opposite the pharynx; adjectives like apical, laminal etc. referring to points of articulation made with the relevant part of the tongue. But, as Ladefoged (1971, p. 37), points out, neither the tongue nor the palate can be conveniently divided into discrete sections, there being no satisfactory points of reference. It is useful, however, to retain a distinction between tip and blade articulations, a parameter which Ladefoged (1971, pp. 38, 93) calls apicality.

In addition to the epithelium and connective tissue there are a number of fibrous septa, which not only may separate some of the tongue muscles, but also serve as sites of attachment for them. These septa also contain in their substance the trunks of some lingual blood vessels and nerves.

The most important of these septa is the median septum (Abd-el-Malek, 1939), which is a fibrous longitudinal partition dividing the tongue into two halves, and giving attachment to the median parts of the transversus muscles, one on either side (cf. Dabelow, 1951, p. 73). It extends from the hyoid bone to the tip being thickest and strongest in its middle portion. In addition to the fibrous septum, there are a number of other connective tissues in the substance of each half of the tongue. The discussion which follows relies heavily on the detailed anatomical studies of Abd-el-Malek (1939) and more recently Miyawaki (1974).

## B. The Muscular System of the Tongue

The tongue muscles on either side of the median septum consist of an intrinsic and an extrinsic group. The extrinsic muscles have their attachments outside the tongue on the hyoid bone, the mandible, and styloid process of the skull, and are capable of altering both the form of the organ and its position in the mouth. The intrinsic muscles, on the other hand, are located entirely within the tongue and so are capable, for the most part, of altering the configuration of the tongue only. It is the intricate interaction of these muscle groups that gives the tongue its great mobility, making it capable of a wide variety of positions and movements. This will become clearer during the discussion on the anatomy and physiology of the different muscles.

The tongue muscles and their general functions are:

1. Intrinsic muscles
   (altering the configuration of the tongue)

   a. longitudinalis superior
   b. longitudinalis inferior
   c. transversus
   d. verticalis

2. Extrinsic muscles
   (altering the position in the mouth and the con-figuration of the tongue)

   a. genioglossus
   b. styloglossus
   c. palatoglossus
   d. hyoglossus

### 1. Muscles Which Alter the Shape of the Tongue—the Intrinsic Muscles

#### a. Longitudinalis Superior

*General description:* The longitudinalis superior is the most superficial muscle of the tongue, lying directly beneath the lamina propria of the dorsum and extending from the root of the tongue to the tip.

*Origin:* The posterior fibres, in the form of a thin sheet, are attached to the mucous membrane of the tongue close to the hyoid bone. Some fibres can be traced back to the epiglottic ligament.

*Course:* The fibres pass in a longitudinal direction throughout the length of the tongue from the root to the tip, thickening to a bulky mass of fibres in the middle (Fig. 24). The fibres course above the transversus and verticalis muscles (Fig. 25). In the vicinity of the root, the fibres travel in a vertical direction.

*Insertion:* The anterior fibres flatten to a thin sheet and are attached to the lamina propria of the mucous membrane at the dorsal part of the tongue tip. Laterally, the fibres spread out to join the longitudinal fibres of the styloglossus, hyoglossus and longitudinalis inferior muscles at the lateral margins of the tongue. There is also probably some interdigitation with fibres of the genioglossus, verticalis and transversus.

*Innervation:* Hypoglossal (twelfth cranial) nerve.

*Function:* Upon contraction, the muscle has the general effect of shortening the tongue, perhaps also making the whole organ wider. In doing

94

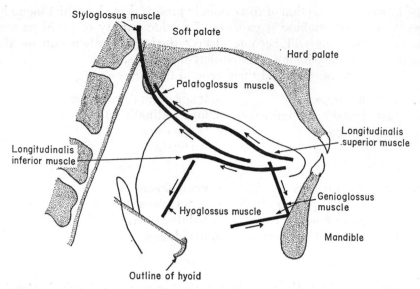

Fig. 24 The movements of the tongue due to contraction of some of the extrinsic and intrinsic tongue muscles.

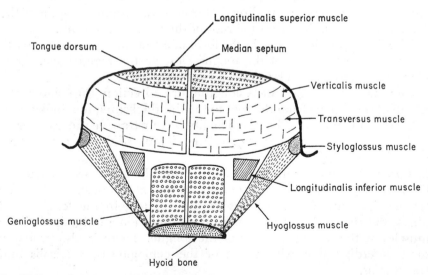

Fig. 25 Coronal section through the tongue showing the positions of the various muscles.

this it probably acts in synergism with the longitudinalis inferior muscle. It is probably also the protagonist muscle in raising the tip for lingual articulations involving contact with the front part of the palate, such as [t], [l], [n] etc. Because this muscle is small and light particularly in the anterior region, it is probably capable of extremely rapid movements. Such movements are necessary, for example, during the articulation of alveolar taps. The lateral fibres may act in synergism with the styloglossus and perhaps also with the palatoglossus (see below) to keep the sides of the tongue raised during articulations requiring a grooved configuration such as [s] and [ʃ]. The most superficial fibres probably act protagonistically in retracting the tip for the articulation of retroflex consonants.

The longitudinalis superior thus acts in conjunction with other intrinsic and extrinsic muscles in altering the shape of the tongue for certain articulations.

### b. Longitudinalis Inferior

*General description:* A paired narrow muscle oval in transverse cross-section, extending longitudinally throughout the length of the tongue in the lateral, ventral part (see Fig. 24).

*Origin:* There are two attachments for this muscle: medial and lateral. The medial fibres decussate with the most lateral and ventral fibres of the genioglossus muscle from the anterior surface of the hyoid bone. The lateral fibres originate at the lateral part of the body of the hyoid bone and the root of the greater cornu of the hyoid where they decussate with the medial fibres of the hyoglossus muscle.

*Course:* The fibres travel longitudinally forwards towards the tip.

*Insertion:* The muscle blends with the anterior fibres of the genioglossus, the hypoglossus, and styloglossus in fixing onto the ventral part of the tip.

*Innervation:* Hypoglossal nerve.

*Function:* The general function of this muscle is probably to pull down and retract the tip. In doing this, it can act in synergism with the anterior fibres of the genioglossus and hyoglossus, with the hyoid fixed by the infrahyoid muscles. This activity is important for the release of stop consonants articulated in the anterior part of the mouth such as [t] and [d]. In pulling down on the tongue tip, the muscle acts as an antagonist to the elevators such as the longitudinalis superior and the styloglossus (see Section II.B.2.b). This activity may be important in producing the finely controlled central groove through which the air is directed during the articulation of [s]. By depressing the tip and probably at the same time bulging the tongue upwards, the main part of the longitudinalis inferior can assist in the formation of the tongue configuration necessary for certain back vowels and velar consonants.

### c. Transversus

*General description:* The transversus muscle forms much of the muscular bulk of the tongue. The fibres are arranged in roughly horizontal layers which fan out laterally toward the tongue margins (see Fig. 25).

*Origin:* The fibres take their origin from the median fibrous septum, and from fibres of the same muscle on the other side particularly in the region of the tip.

*Course:* From the median septum, the fibres course laterally on either side of the tongue between the longitudinalis superior muscle dorsally, and the genioglossus and longitudinalis inferior ventrally (Fig. 25). Some of the superficial fibres travel in a dorso-lateral direction toward the tongue margins.

*Insertion:* The longer fibres of the muscle reach the lamina propria of the mucous membrane of the sides of the tongue. The majority of fibres decussate with neighbouring muscles such as the verticalis and genioglossus. In the tip region the fibres interdigitate with the longitudinalis superior and longitudinalis inferior and also perhaps some fibres of styloglossus and hyoglossus.

*Innervation:* Hypoglossal nerve.

*Function:* Upon contraction, the transversus fibres, particularly the more superficial fibres, draw the edges of the tongue upwards, and by compressing the width of the tongue, may help to elongate it longitudinally. It thus acts mainly in synergism with other muscles such as the styloglossus, which inserts along the tongue margins, in forming a central groove in the tip and blade for certain fricative articulations particularly [s] and [ʃ]. Together with the posterior part of the genioglossus, it may help to push forward the tongue for frontal articulations such as alveolar stops and fricatives, when preceded, for instance, by a low back vowel.

   The muscle also probably acts as an antagonist muscle to the verticalis and hyoglossus in achieving finely graded tongue configurations such as the grooved configuration necessary for the articulation of [s].

### d. Verticalis

*General description:* The muscle consists of several bundles of short fibres placed more or less in a vertical direction. The fibres decussate with the transversus fibres thus forming a considerable part of the central body of the tongue (Fig. 25).

*Origin:* Most of the fibres originate in the mucosa of the dorsum. The greatest concentration of fibres occurs in the middle portion of the tongue immediately adjacent to the median septum.

*Course:* Vertically downwards on either side of the median septum.

*Insertion:* Most of the fibres insert into the sub-mucous membrane on the inferior surface of the tongue. Some of the shorter fibres interdigitate with other muscles particularly the transversus and the longitudinalis inferior.

*Innervation:* Hypoglossal nerve.

*Function:* The general function of the muscle is probably to narrow the vertical cross-section of the tongue and flatten it out sideways. In flattening the tongue the muscle probably plays an important part in the production of front vowels such as [i], and in pushing the tongue out laterally to maintain palatal contact for the closure phase in alveolar and palatal stops. This activity is also important to maintain a lateral seal between the upper and lower teeth during production of the fricative [s].

The median fibres of the transversus may conceivably act independently of the rest of the muscle in forming a grooved configuration in the tongue's dorsum. Synergistic contraction of the styloglossus, palatoglossus and transversus will contribute to this grooved configuration.

## 2. Muscles that Primarily Alter the Position of the Tongue in the Mouth—the Extrinsic Muscles

### a. Genioglossus

The origin, course and insertion of the genioglossus has already been discussed above in Chapter 4 under the suprahyoid muscle group. The muscle is, however, properly regarded as a muscle of the tongue so its function in altering the position, and to a certain extent the shape of the tongue, will be discussed here.

*Function:* The anterior fibres contract to retract and depress the tip (Fig. 24). Here the muscle acts in synergism with other retractors and lowerers of the tongue tip such as the longitudinalis inferior, in the release of alveolar stop consonants. The posterior fibres of the genioglossus contract to draw the tongue forwards in the mouth while the mandible remains fixed. This will result in the whole body of the tongue moving forward in the mouth. This anterior movement of the tongue is important for virtually all articulations made in the front part of the mouth particularly when they are preceded by a velar articulation. Also, with the help of tongue elevators such as the styloglossus and palatoglossus, the posterior fibres of the genioglossus will cause the tongue body to move upwards and forwards in the mouth. The intermediate fibres of the genioglossus act with the posterior fibres to draw the tongue forward and perhaps depress the middle of the tongue.

Because the posterior and anterior fibres of the genioglossus independently serve different functions (MacNeilage and Sholes, 1964, pp. 227–228), it is perhaps possible to regard the genioglossus as comprising two different muscles.

### b. Styloglossus

*General description:* The paired styloglossus muscle is a flat, narrow, fan-shaped sheet of fibres which travels downwards towards the tongue from the styloid process of the temporal bone.

*Origin:* The muscle begins as a short slip of fibres arising from the anterior surface of the styloid process in front of the ear.

*Course:* Just anterior to its origin, the fibres begin to radiate slightly as they course downwards and anteriorly. Before the fibres reach the tongue they divide into two parts—an upper and a lower part.

*Insertion:* The lower fibres decussate with the lateral surface of the hyoglossus muscle (Fig. 25). The upper fibres constitute the longer part, and they travel along the margins of the tongue towards the tip where they interdigitate with the fibres of the longitudinalis inferior muscle. Some isolated fibres probably reach the tip.

*Innervation:* Hypoglossal nerve.

*Function:* The styloglossus is probably one of the principal elevators of the tongue. It may act in synergism to the posterior part of the genioglossus in elevating the tongue for velar articulations such as [k], [g]. The antagonistic muscles to this activity would be principally the hyoglossus acting from a fixed hyoid bone. The co-ordinated activity between the styloglossus and hyoglossus presumably places the tongue in the appropriate position for the production of most vowels.

Because its insertion is primarily along the edges of the tongue (Fig. 25), contraction of the styloglossus may tend to raise the lateral margins so forming a cup-shaped configuration or sulcalization towards the back part of the tongue. This sulcalization occurs during articulation of [s] and [ʃ]. To prevent sulcalization of the back part of the tongue during some articulations such as velar stops, the longitudinalis inferior probably acts as a synergist in bulging the tongue upwards.

## c. Palatoglossus

*General description:* The paired palatoglossus is usually described as a depressor of the velum (Kaplan, 1971). It does, however, insert into the tongue so it can be regarded as one of the extrinsic tongue muscles. It is sometimes referred to as the glossopalatinus.

*Origin:* The fibres originate from the under surface of the velum, where they spread out to interdigitate with those fibres from the opposite side. It forms the lowest muscular stratum of the velum.

*Course:* The fibres course downwards and laterally (Fig. 24) forming the anterior pillars of the fauces in front of the tonsil. Diamond (1952) notes that the palatoglossus probably forms a more or less circular sphincter because its fibres blend both in the tongue itself and in the soft palate.

*Insertion:* Most of the fibres interdigitate with the transversus fibres and the superficial fibres of the styloglossus and hyoglossus, at the edges of the tongue.

*Innervation:* Probably the vagus (tenth cranial) nerve, through the pharyngeal plexus.

*Function:* When the velum is fixed, the palatoglossus muscle can assist in raising the back part of the tongue. It thus acts here in synergism with the styloglossus and in antagonism to the hyoglossus muscle. Together with the styloglossus and some intrinsic muscles, particularly the longitudinalis inferior, it can help bulge the back of the tongue upwards for velar articulations. As the muscle inserts into the sides of the tongue, it is possible that it contributes also to sulcalization of the back part of the tongue.

Because the muscle forms a link between the body of the tongue and the velum, movements of the tongue may to some extent influence the position of the velum. A low tongue movement, for example, will draw down on the velum because of the mechanical linkage, so opening the passage into the nasal cavity (Moll, 1962; Moll and Shriner, 1967). This may result in a greater tendency to nasalization when the tongue is in a low position.

## d. Hyoglossus

The hyoglossus muscle has already been discussed in Chapter 4 as one of the elevators of the hyoid bone. Because it inserts into the tongue, however, it has some function in changing that organ's position in the mouth. When the hyoid bone is fixed, the hyoglossus can function as the main lowerer of the tongue. The anterior fibres act with the anterior fibres of the genioglossus and the longitudinalis interior in retracting and lowering the tongue tip for the release of certain articulations.

The posterior fibres are inserted into the lateral part of the body of the tongue so contraction will tend to pull down on the sides. These fibres thus act as the main antagonists for the styloglossus and palatoglossus (when acting from a fixed velum), and contribute to the production of delicate surface adjustments necessary for certain grooved fricatives such as [s], [ʃ].

It may also work in conjunction with the styloglossus in positioning the tongue body for the production of back vowels (MacNeilage and Sholes, 1964, p. 228). One would expect therefore the tongue to have a convex configuration (with respect to the palate) during vowel articulation. The anterior fibres probably oppose the forward action of the posterior part of the genioglossus in achieving a balanced control of the tongue body for the production of most front vowels.

## C. Articulatory Parameters of Lingual Activity

The functions of the various tongue muscles in producing the wide range of different lingual postures and configurations during speech can be summarized under seven articulatory parameters. These parameters, which aim at defining all the known tongue shapes and motions used during speech production are compiled on the basis of the anatomical and physiological outline above and information from experimental techniques such as palatography (both direct palatography and electro-palatography) and radiography (Hardcastle, 1974).

The seven articulatory parameters for specifying the different lingual motions and configurations during speech are illustrated schematically in Figs. 26–29. They are:

1. Horizontal forward–backward movement of the tongue body
2. Vertical upwards–downwards movement of the tongue body
3. Horizontal forward–backward movement of the tip–blade
4. Vertical upwards–downwards movement of the tip–blade
5. Transverse cross-sectional configuration of the tongue body: convex–concave, in relation to the palate
6. Transverse cross-sectional configuration extending throughout the whole length of the tongue, particularly the tip and blade—degree of central grooving
7. Surface plan of the tongue dorsum—spread, tapered.

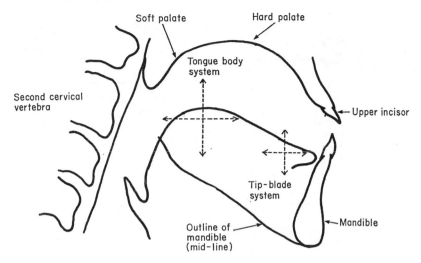

Fig. 26 Sagittal view of the tongue illustrating the lingual articulatory parameters 1–4.

Movements of the tongue body are described in relation to a fixed point within the body of the tongue. The point chosen was the reference point sometimes used in X-ray measurements of lingual dimensions (e.g. Wildman, 1961) and is defined as the intersection of a line drawn from the tip of the lower incisor to the centre of the second cervical vertebra and another line drawn vertically from the junction between the hard and the soft palates. The boundary of the tip–blade is fixed arbitrarily as the point on the tongue dorsum opposite the junction between the

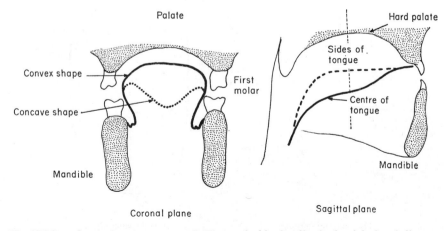

Fig. 27 Lingual articulatory parameter 5. The vertical broken line in the right-hand diagram shows the point where the coronal plane section is taken.

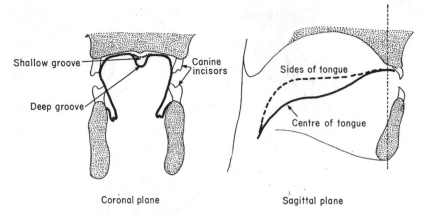

Fig. 28 Lingual articulatory parameter 6. On the right the vertical broken line shows the point at which the coronal plane section was taken.

alveolar ridge and the hard palate when the tongue is in a position for the articulation of [ə].

Different articulatory movements and configurations can be achieved by combinations of these seven basic parameters. Thus vowels utilize primarily parameters 1 and 2, while alveolar stop consonants utilize parameters 1, 2, 3, 4, and 7. Grooved fricatives such as [s] require maximal participation of all articulatory parameters.

The muscular systems responsible for these parameters will now be specified.

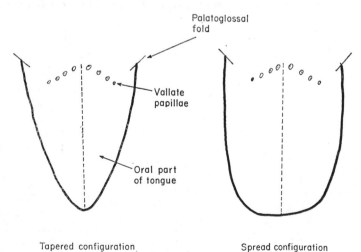

Fig. 29 Lingual articulatory parameter 7.

## 1. Forward–Backward Movement of the Tongue Body

Forward movement of the tongue body is accomplished primarily by the posterior part of the genioglossus, when contracting from a fixed mandible. The synergist muscles in this activity are probably the anterior suprahyoid muscles. The hyoid bone is tilted forward by balanced contraction between the anterior infrahyoid muscles (the sternohyoideus and omohyoideus) and the stylohyoideus. The forward movement is usually accompanied by an upward tongue body movement.

The horizontal backward movement is accomplished primarily by the styloglossus and constrictor pharyngis medius (see Chapter 4, Section III.A.1.*g*). The upward tendency of the styloglossus could be opposed by the thyrohyoideus (see Chapter 4, Section III.A.2) pulling down on the cornu of the hyoid bone. A horizontal backward movement of the tongue probably only occurs in pharyngeal articulations, for example Arabic [ħ], and also to some extent in low back vowels such as [ɒ]. The backward movement is frequently combined with an upward movement in the production of velar and uvular articulations such as [x], etc.

## 2. Upward–Downward Movement of the Tongue Body

The vertical upward movement of the tongue body is carried out by the styloglossus and the palatoglossus (only if the velum is fixed by the levator and tensor muscles), with the longitudinalis inferior acting in synergism. Any unwanted backward movement could be opposed by the forward pull of the posterior genioglossus.

The upward movement of the body may be important for some close central vowels such as [ɨ] and for palatal consonants such as palatal clicks and stops.

The protagonist muscle in the downward movement of the tongue body is the hyoglossus muscle. In lowering the tongue the infrahyoid musculature (Chapter 4, Section III.A.2) plays a synergist role. In addition, the intermediate fibres of the genioglossus may play some part in depressing the tongue body, particularly the centre of the tongue, when contracting from a fixed mandible.

The downward movement would be particularly important for vowel production where a balanced contraction between the elevators and depressors of the tongue is necessary to give the specific configuration appropriate for each vowel. The downward movement would also be important for the release phase of most stops and fricatives. For alveolar articulation, however, the tip–blade parameters may be functionally more significant.

## 3. Forward–Backward Movement of the Tip–Blade

Protrusion of the tongue tip is achieved primarily by the intrinsic transversus muscle acting in synergism with the posterior genioglossus. This movement usually involves parameter 1 as well.

A backward movement of the tip is accomplished by both intrinsic longitudinal muscles contracting simultaneously, thus retracting the tip "into" the body of the tongue. A backward movement of the tip is important in retroflex articulations. Here, however, the situation is rather complex as the tip must also be extended slightly to facilitate the curled backward movement. At the same time as the tip moves backward, the body is depressed, probably by the hyoglossus.

## 4. Upward–Downward Movement of the Tip–Blade

In raising the tip–blade the protagonist muscle is the longitudinalis superior. This movement can be largely independent of tongue body movement so double articulations are possible. Upward movement of the tip is often accompanied by a general forward upward movement of the tongue body (parameters 1 and 2), for example approaching the closure phase of an alveolar stop [t] in the environment [a t i]. However, when the body is already positioned by the extrinsic musculature in a close front position (e.g. for [i]), the upward movement of the tip for a [t] is largely independent of the tongue body movement.

The downward movement of the tip–blade is accomplished by both the longitudinalis inferior and the anterior part of the genioglossus when acting from a fixed mandible. As with the upward movement, the tip–blade may here act independently of the tongue body. The downward movement can be part of the release phase of alveolar articulations such as [t], [l], [n]; it can also provide balanced control of the central groove in the tip for the fricative [s]. Here it acts antagonistically to elevators such as the longitudinalis superior, styloglossus, and palatoglossus.

## 5. Concave–Convex Cross-sectional Configuration

The protagonist muscles contributing to a concave configuration are the styloglossus, palatoglossus and transversus. Because the insertion of the styloglossus is mainly in the posterior margins of the tongue, and because this muscle is probably the largest and strongest of the three, the concave configuration occurs frequently in the posterior part of the tongue. X-ray photographs made of the tongue during articulation of [s] show clearly a wide concave configuration in the back of the tongue (Hardcastle, 1974).

The convex configuration is produced primarily by the hyoglossus which inserts into the lateral margins of the tongue. When contracting in conjunction with the longitudinalis inferior muscle during the production of velar and palatal stops, the resulting bulging backwards of the tongue will tend to have a convex configuration making an airtight seal with the palate. As mentioned earlier, the tongue is positioned for vowel articulation by the balanced contraction of the elevators (styloglossus, palatoglossus) and the depressors (hyoglossus, infrahyoid musculature). In some cases this may produce a convex configuration for the vowel.

## 6. Degree of Central Grooving

The production of an accurately controlled central groove in the anterior part of the tongue, such as occurs during the articulation of [s] requires the co-operation of many muscles, and is probably the most complex configuration that takes place during speech.

The muscles probably most directly responsible for the central groove are the transversus (median part) and the verticalis muscle (particularly the superficial fibres). The tongue may be spread out slightly by the whole verticalis. At the same time the styloglossus and palatoglossus (from a fixed velum) may act synergistically with the transversus in keeping the sides raised. In the articulation of [s] this lateral movement has the effect of bracing the sides of the tongue against the teeth.

If the grooving occurs in the tip-blade, the central part of the tip is depressed by both the longitudinalis inferior and the anterior part of the genioglossus, when acting from a fixed mandible. Antagonistic contraction of the longitudinalis superior would determine the depth of the groove, more tension probably creating a shallower groove.

## 7. Spread-tapered Surface Plan Configuration

The spread configuration is accomplished primarily by contraction of the verticalis muscle which tends to narrow the thickness of the tongue and spread it out sideways. This spreading is important for stop articulation in obstructing the air-flow by pressing the tongue against the palate. Thus for an alveolar stop, e.g. [t], contact is seen on a palatogram as covering a horseshoe-shaped area of the palate including the alveolar ridge region and along both sides of the teeth and gums. In the articulation of [s] the spreading action is important in producing the lateral seal between the teeth and gums, so directing the airflow through the controlled central goove (cf. Lawson and Bond, 1968, p. 115). For some vowel articulations such as [i], [e], considerable contact is also made along both sides of the palate up to the alveolar region. The tip is here lowered allowing the passage of air over the central line of the tongue.

The tapered configuration is produced by the narrowing effect of the transversus muscle. The superficial fibres will tend to pull the sides of the tongue inwards, an action which could be opposed by the hyoglossus. If the hyoglossus does exert its downward pull on the sides of the tongue, the configuration of the tongue will not only be tapered but will have a convex configuration, particularly if the hyoglossus contraction is stronger than the transversus.

The tapering often accompanies a protrusion of the tongue or raising of the tip. When the tongue tip is raised as it may be for instance in a dental articulation of [l] by some speakers, the tapering of the tip may be accompanied by contraction of the posterior part of the genioglossus and the longitudinalis superior.

# III. Physiology of Mandibular Movements

## A. General Description of the Mandible

The mandible is intimately connected to both the hyoid bone and the tongue by means of muscles, so any movement it makes will usually alter both the position and, to a lesser extent, the shape of the tongue. When viewed from above the mandible is a roughly U-shaped arch. The closed end of the arch is situated anteriorly and constitutes the area of the chin. At both open ends of the U, bony extensions (rami) run upwards to join with the temporal bones in front of the ear at the temporomandibular joints. Figure 30 shows a lateral view of the mandible with the various structural parts marked, and the directions of movement of the mandible under the influence of the various mandibular muscles.

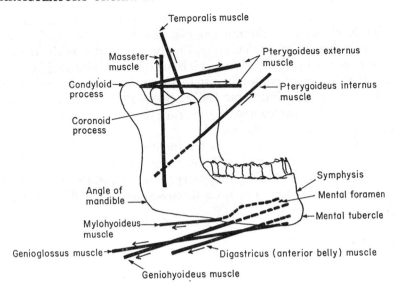

Fig. 30 Lateral view of mandible showing the main structural parts and the movements of the mandible when the various mandibular muscles contract from fixed origins.

## B. The Mandibular Muscular System

The main movements of the mandible and the muscular groups contributing to these movements are as follows:

1. Raising:
   a. pterygoideus internus
   b. masseter
   c. temporalis

2. Lowering:
   a. pterygoideus externus
   b. geniohyoideus
   c. digastricus (anterior belly)
   d. mylohyoideus
   e. genioglossus

3. Protrusion:
   a. pterygoideus externus
   b. pterygoideus internus

4. Retraction:
   a. temporalis (posterior fibres)
   b. mylohyoideus
   c. geniohyoideus
   d. digastricus (anterior belly)
   e. genioglossus

5. Oblique lateral movement:
   a. pterygoideus externus
   b. temporalis (posterior fibres)

All of these movements are particularly important for chewing and grinding food. Some of the movements, however, are also of some importance during speech articulation. Firstly, any raising of the mandible will also raise the hyoid bone, unless it is fixed by the infrahyoid musculature, and this movement will assist in the production, for instance, of close front vowels (Lindblom, 1967). Secondly, any lowering of the mandible will alter the volume in the oral cavity thus having some effect on the oral resonance of the sound.

Most of the mandibular muscles mentioned above have already been described under muscles of the tongue and hyoid. Some of the muscles, however, including the pterygoideus muscles, the masseter, and the temporalis have not been discussed so they will be described fully.

## 1. Muscles of Elevation

### a. Pterygoideus Internus

*General description:* The pterygoideus internus is a thick, quadrilateral muscle lying mostly on the medial surface of the mandibular ramus.
*Origin:* Most of the fibres originate on the pterygoid fossa of the sphenoid bone of the skull. The innermost fibres originate from the medial surface of the lateral pterygoid plate.
*Course:* The fibres run posteriorly and downward (see Fig. 30).
*Insertion:* Most fibres insert at the rear of the ramus of the mandible.
*Innervation:* Internal pterygoideus nerve branch of the mandibular nerve, part of the trigeminal (fifth cranial) nerve complex.
*Function:* The main function is to work in synergism with the masseter and temporalis in raising the mandible. It can also help to protrude the lower part of the mandible because of its slightly posterior course. This movement will oppose the natural tendency to move backward when raised because of the nature of the temporomandibular joint. The muscle also acts in antagonism to the anterior suprahyoid muscles in obtaining the balance of lip position necessary for production of the labiodental fricatives [f], [v]. The raising, protruding movement is probably important in achieving the correct relationship between the upper and lower jaws during production of [s].

### b. Masseter

*General description:* The masseter is the most superficial of the mandibular elevators. It is a thick, flat, quadrilateral muscle lying on the outer surface of the ramus.

*Origin:* The zygomatic arch of the maxilla bone.
*Course:* Downward.
*Insertion:* The angle and ramus of the mandible covering a large area.
*Innervation:* Masseter branch of the mandibular nerve.
*Function:* Because of its relatively massive size, the masseter is probably the most powerful mandibular muscle. In closing the mandible and putting pressure on the molar teeth it is undoubtedly one of the most important muscles of mastication.

The functions of the muscle during speech are probably similar to those of the pterygoideus internus in elevating the mandible and so the tongue, for example during the production of alveolar articulations.

### c. Temporalis

*General description:* A large, paired, triangular sheet of fibres covering a wide area on the side of the skull.
*Origin:* The fibres arise from a large area of the skull extending from the side of the forehead to behind the ear.
*Course:* The fibres course downwards and anteriorly, converging near their insertion.
*Insertion:* The fibres insert upon the coronoid process of the ramus of the mandible.
*Innervation:* The temporalis branch of the mandibluar nerve.
*Function:* The muscle acts in synergism with the masseter and pterygoideus internus in elevating the mandible. The posterior fibres also probably help to retract the mandible slightly (Fig. 30). This retraction is assisted by the backward pull of the anterior suprahyoid muscles (see Chapter 4, Section III.A.1). The infrahyoid musculature act as fixators keeping the hyoid bone steady for this movement.

As with the other elevators, this muscle acts in antagonism to the mandibular depressors in maintaining the balanced position necessary for the production of some fricatives such as [f], [s] and most front vowels.

## 2. Muscles of Depression

### a. Pterygoideus Externus

*General description:* The pterygoideus externus is a thick, triangular muscle located deep to the temporalis.
*Origin:* The fibres take their origin from two heads. The larger, inferior

head arises from the lateral pterygoid plate, and the smaller, superior head from the greater wing of the sphenoid bone of the skull.

*Course:* Fibres from the two heads interdigitate with each other as they pass posteriorly and horizontally in front of the temporomandibular joint.

*Insertion:* The condyloid process of the mandible and also the temporomandibular joint itself.

*Innervation:* The pterygoideus branch of the mandibular nerve.

*Function:* As the fibres travel in a more or less horizontal direction, the muscle acts more to protrude the mandible than to depress it. However, acting in synergism with the other depressors, it assists in the lowering movements. Van Riper and Irwin (1958, p. 356) note that the forward movement may be important during articulation of [s], particularly if the person's jaw is small.

The muscle also assists in the oblique lateral movements important for grinding food, by functioning alternatively with the posterior fibres of the temporalis.

### b. c. d. and e. Anterior Suprahyoid Musculature

These muscles have already been described in detail elsewhere (Chapter 4, Section III.A.1). When the infrahyoids fix the hyoid bone they may function to depress the mandible. It is only when the position of the mandible is fixed by contraction of the mandibular elevators, that contraction of the suprahyoids will result in an upward, forward movement of the hyoid bone.

The mandibular depressors are important for the rapid lowering of the mandible, for instance in facilitating the release of the closure for stops. Also they may act antagonistically to the elevators of the mandible in achieving an optimal mandibular position for the articulation of vowels.

### 3. Muscles of Protrusion

The primary protruder of the mandible is the pterygoideus externus described above under muscles of depression. The pterygoideus internus and the superficial part of the masseter may act synergistically to assist the forward movement.

The protrusion movement may be important, for instance, in the articulation of labiodental frication such as [f] in some peoples' articulation, and bilabial fricatives such as [Φ]. Also, as was mentioned above, the protrusion movement may aid the articulation of [s].

## 4. Muscles of Retraction

The principal retracting muscles are the suprahyoid muscles mentioned above, assisted by the posterior fibres of the temporalis muscle. The retracting movement will usually be accompanied by a lowering of the mandible, although the temporalis may prevent this to some extent.

The movement is sometimes seen in the production of open back vowels but the amount of retraction in speech is probably only slight.

## 5. Muscles that Produce an Oblique Lateral Movement

The protagonist muscles for the lateral, grinding movement of the mandible are the pterygoideus externus and temporalis (posterior fibres). The movement is important for grinding and chewing food and is brought about by alternate protrusion and retraction of each side of the mandible with activity by the elevating muscles. The two protagonist muscles function alternatively and are assisted synergistically by all the mandibular muscles mentioned above.

The grinding and chewing movement is probably not of great importance in speech production (Van Riper and Irwin, 1958, p. 363). However, some individuals, who have asymmetric jaw movements as idiosyncrasies, may use this grinding movement in speech.

# IV. Physiology of Lip Movements

## A. General Description of the Lips

The lips encircle the mouth orifice as a pair of fleshy folds composed largely of tissue, blood vessels, glands, nerves and muscle. The skin of the lips terminates at a sharp demarcation line, the vermilion border, visible as the boundary of the red-hued part of the lips.

Anatomically, the lips have a rather complex structure. The most characteristic feature is a large sphincter muscle, the orbicularis oris, which constitutes the main muscular part of the lips. A large number of facial and other muscles from virtually all directions interdigitate with the fibres of the orbicularis oris, thus allowing the lips a great versatility of movement. Many of the delicate lip movements serve primarily an expressive function; however, many postures and configurations of the lips are important for speech articulation, for example, in the production of labial stops and fricatives, and rounded vowels such as [u], [y] etc.

Because of their relative accessibility, the lips have been the subject of extensive electromyographic research (Harris *et al.*, 1965; Öhman, 1967; Fromkin, 1966; MacNeilage and De Clerk, 1969; Tatham and Morton, 1972). The underlying aim of much of this research, particularly by the Haskins group, has been to determinate whether there are invariances in the motor commands to the obicularis oris and other lip muscles, during the articulation of labial stops such as [p], [b] in various phonetic contexts. The results have not, however, been very conclusive.

Except for the orbicularis oris muscle, which is common to both, the upper and lower lips are supplied largely by separate muscles and can move independently. The lower lip is more mobile than the upper lip, probably because its position is affected by any movements of the mandible. In fact the opening action of the lips, for example, in the release phase of bilabial stops, is preceded usually by a lowering of the mandible (Fujimura, 1961, p. 240).

Movements of the upper lip are particularly important in producing facial expressions associated with emotions such as disdain, contempt, surprise, etc. (Kaplan, 1971, p. 386).

## B. Muscles of the Lips

The main movements of the lips, and the muscles responsible for these movements are illustrated schematically in Fig. 31. They are:

| | |
|---|---|
| 1. Closing lips: | *a.* orbicularis oris |
| 2. Raising upper lip: | *a.* zygomaticus minor |
| | *b.* levator labii superior |
| | *c.* levator labii superior alaeque nasi |
| 3. Lowering bottom lip: | *a.* depressor labii inferior |
| 4. Rounding lips: | *a.* orbicularis oris |
| 5. Protruding lips: | *a.* mentalis (lower lip) |
| | *b.* orbicularis oris (deeper fibres) |
| 6. Retracting angle of mouth: | *a.* buccinator |
| | *b.* zygomaticus major |
| | *c.* risorius |
| 7. Raising angles of mouth: | *a.* levator anguli oris |
| | *b.* zygomaticus major |

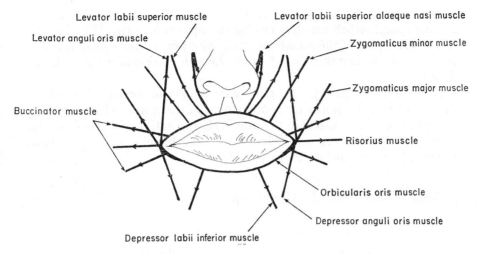

Fig. 31 Some of the possible movements of the lips under the influence of the main labial muscles.

8. Lowering angles of mouth:   *a.* depressor anguli oris
                               *b.* platysma

## 1. Muscles that Close the Lips

### *a. Orbicularis Oris*

*General description:* A large sphincter muscle encircling the lips and making up most of the muscular part of the lips. The muscle can be regarded as being comprised mainly of the interlacing fibres of muscles that converge upon the lips. The upper and lower fibres of the muscle meet at the angles of the mouth.

*Origin, course, and insertion:* The fibres encircle the lips joining at the angles of the mouth. It is frequently extemely difficult to separate the fibres of the orbicularis oris from the superficial fibres of the faeial muscles.

*Innervation:* The facial (seventh cranial) nerve.

*Function:* The main function of the muscle is to adduct the lips, often pressing them against the teeth when contracting strongly. It achieves this by drawing the upper lip down and the lower lip up. The activity in drawing the lower lip up is probably assisted by elevators of the mandible such as the masseter, temporalis, and the pterygoideus internus (see Section III) as well as the inferior fibres of the levator anguli oris (see Section IV.B.7). This adduction activity is important for any sound which involves closing the lips such as [p], [b], [m] etc. The inferior part of the muscle probably also plays some role in pressing the lower lip against the upper teeth in the articulation of the labiodental fricative [f].

Activity of the muscle can also cause puckering or rounding of the lips because of the sphincter arrangement of the fibres. This puckering of the lips may be avoided in the simple closing activity by simultaneous contraction of retracting muscles such as the buccinator, zygomaticus major, platysma, and risorius (see below).

## 2. Muscles that Raise the Upper Lip

### a. Zygomaticus Minor

*General description:* This muscle is sometimes called the zygomatic head of the quadratus labii superior. Here it will be regarded as a separate muscle.

*Origin:* The fibres arise from the facial surface of the zygomatic bone of the skull (Fig. 32).

*Course:* Downwards and slightly medially.

*Insertion:* Skin of the upper lip and the orbicularis oris muscle (see Fig. 31) just lateral to the mid-line.

*Innervation:* Facial (seventh cranial) nerve.

*Function:* The protagonist function of the muscle is to raise the upper lip. This activity may be important during the articulation of [f] by elevating the upper lip slightly to allow the air to flow through the stricture made by the lower lip against the upper teeth. The synergist muscles in this activity would probably be the retractors of the lips such as the buccinator, zygomaticus major and the muscles which raise the angles of the mouth, particularly the levator anguli oris (Section IV.B.7).

### b. Levator Labii Superior

*General description:* This muscle is also called the infraorbital head of the quadratus labii superior.

*Origin:* The maxilla bone of the skull immediately above the infraorbital foramen (see Fig. 32).

*Course:* Downwards.

*Insertion:* The fibres are inserted into the skin of the nasolabial groove.

*Innervation:* Facial (seventh cranial) nerve.

*Function:* The main function of the muscle is to raise the upper lip particularly the middle region. It acts as a synergist to the zygomaticus minor in the production of [f].

### c. Levator Labii Superior Alaeque Nasi

*General description:* Also called the angular head of the quadratus labii superior muscle. The muscle consists of a narrow band of fibres.
*Origin:* Frontal process of the maxilla bone.
*Course:* Downwards and laterally along the sides of the nose.
*Insertion:* Partly into the wings of the nose and partly into the naso-labial groove where some fibres interdigitate with the orbicularis oris.
*Innervation:* Facial (seventh cranial) nerve.
*Function:* The muscle can raise the middle part of the upper lip and elevate the wings of the nose. It can act synergistically to the zygomaticus minor and the levator labii superior as mentioned above.

## 3. Muscles which Lower the Lower Lip

### a. Depressor Labii Inferior

*General description:* A small, flat, quadrangular muscle situated beneath the lower lip.
*Origin:* The outer surface of the mandible between the mental foramen and the symphysis (Fig. 32).
*Course:* Upwards and medially, the fibres travelling deep to the depressor anguli oris.
*Insertion:* Most of the fibres insert into the orbicularis oris, and the skin of the lower lip.
*Innervation:* Facial (seventh cranial) nerve.
*Function:* The muscle is the main depressor of the lower lip. It is thus important for the release of bilabial stop consonants such as [p], [b]. This activity is assisted probably by the muscles which depress the mandible such as the anterior suprahyoid muscles (see Chapter 4, Section III.A.1).

## 4. Muscles that Round the Lips

### a. Orbicularis Oris

The orbicularis oris has already been described above under Section IV.B.1.*a.* In its sphincter activity it can round the lips for the production of rounded vowels such as [u], [y] etc. (Öhman *et al.*, 1965, p. 3).

Different degrees of rounding are probably produced by different degrees of tension in the muscle, and by elevation or depression of the mandible, thus moving the lower lip towards or away from the upper lip. The lips may not necessarily be protruded during the rounding. They may be restrained by the principal retractor muscles, the buccinator, zygomaticus major, and the risorius (see Section IV.B.6).

## 5. Muscles that Protrude the Lips

### a. Mentalis

*General description:* The mentalis muscle consists of a paired small bundle of fibres situated in the chin.
*Origin:* The mandible just below the incisor teeth (Fig. 32).
*Course:* Downward.
*Insertion:* The fibres insert into the skin of the chin.
*Innervation:* Facial (seventh cranial) nerve.
*Function:* The main activity of the muscle is to draw the skin of the chin and lower lip upwards. This has the effect of everting the lower lip and protruding it slightly. When contracting simultaneously with the orbicularis oris, a protruded, rounded configuration for close rounded vowels such as [u], [y] can be produced. The muscle may also act as a synergist to the orbicularis oris in closing the lips by drawing up the lower lip.

### b. Orbicularis Oris

The muscle has already been discussed above. Another possible function that the muscle (particularly the deeper fibres) fulfils is to act with the mentalis in protruding the lips. This is basically the sphincter activity of the muscle mentioned above under Section IV.B.1. For more open rounded vowels such as [ɸ] and [ɔ], the lips are probably abducted by muscles such as the zygomaticus minor, levator labii superior, and levator labii superior alaeque nasi raising the upper lip, and the depressor labii inferior lowering the lower lip. Balanced contraction between these muscles and a specific setting of the mandible probably contribute to achieving the appropriate configuration for the rounded vowels.

## 6. Muscles that Retract the Angle of the Mouth

### a. Buccinator

*General description:* The buccinator muscle is so called because it is the main muscle used in playing the bugle. It is a large powerful muscle regarded as one of the main muscles of the cheek.

*Origin:* Most of the fibres arise from the pterygomandibular raphe, which is a tendinous link between the internal pterygoid plate on the skull, and the mandible, near the back molars. Some fibres of the constrictor pharyngis superior (see Chapter 4, Section III.A.1.*g*) are attached to this raphe. Other fibres of the buccinator arise from the lateral surfaces of the mandible and the maxilla opposite the sockets of the molar teeth.

*Course:* Forward towards the angles of the mouth, parallel to the risorius (see Section IV.B.6.*c*). Some fibres course medially.

*Insertion:* The fibres enter the angles of the mouth and extend as far as the upper and lower lips (see Fig. 31). Many of the fibres decussate at the angle of the mouth.

*Innervation:* Facial (seventh cranial) nerve.

*Function:* The main function is to retract the angles of the mouth perhaps compressing the lips against the teeth. This activity is antagonistic to the protruding action of the orbicularis oris and mentalis muscles. The muscle is probably active as a synergist to the lower fibres of the orbicularis oris, the zygomaticus major, the depressor anguli oris, the risorius, and the platysma (see below) in drawing back the angles of the mouth and the lower lip during articulation of [f], and "spread" vowels such as [i], [e]. The muscle is probably also the protagonist in the production of bilabial fricatives such as [Φ].

### b. Zygomaticus Major

*General description:* The zygomaticus major is a long, slender, oblong-shaped muscle lying superficial to the maxillary bone.

*Origin:* Outer surface of zygomatic bone (see Fig. 32).

*Course:* Downwards and medially.

*Insertion:* The fibres insert into the angles of the mouth, into the orbicularis oris muscle and the skin of the lips.

*Innervation:* Facial (seventh cranial) nerve.

*Function:* The main function is to draw the corners of the mouth laterally and slightly upwards. The upwards motion is synergistic to that of the levator anguli oris and is probably important in the production of [f] and in the articulation of spread vowels such as [i], [e] etc. The muscle may also function with the risorius in drawing the angles of the mouth laterally in achieving the appropriate configuration for [s].

### c. Risorius

*General description:* A flat, superficially placed muscle lateral to the lips.

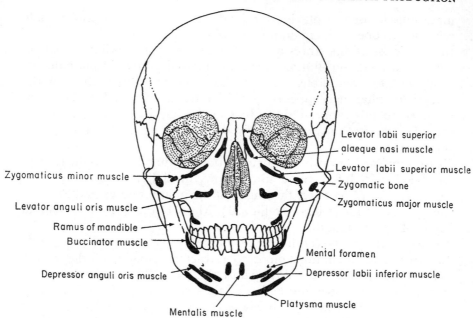

Fig. 32 Frontal view of skull showing the points of attachment of the main labial muscles (after Cunningham, 1964).

It can perhaps be regarded as a continuation of the platysma muscle on the face.

*Origin:* The fibres arise from the fascia over the masseter muscle on the outer rami of the mandible.

*Course:* Horizontal and forwards toward the angle of the mouth.

*Insertion:* The skin and mucosa of the upper lip and the mucosa just lateral to the angle of the mouth. A few fibres also insert into the lower lip.

*Innervation:* Facial (seventh cranial) nerve.

*Function:* The muscle functions mainly to draw the angles of the mouth laterally and so help to spread the lips in the production of [s] and spread vowels such as [i], [e]. The muscle also probably acts synergistically to the buccinator and zygomaticus major in retracting the angles of the mouth during articulation of [f] and [Φ].

7. Muscles that Raise the Angles of the Mouth

*a. Levator Anguli Oris*

*General description:* The muscle is also known as the caninus. It is a flat triangular muscle.

*Origin:* The surface of the maxilla bone just below the infraorbital foramen (Fig. 32).
*Course:* Downwards and slightly laterally.
*Insertion:* Most fibres insert into the orbicularis oris near the angle of the mouth. Some fibres reach the lower lip.
*Innervation:* Facial (seventh cranial) nerve.
*Function:* The main function of the muscle is to elevate the angles of the mouth and the upper lip. Because of the insertion of some fibres into the lower lip it is possible that the muscle acts also to raise the lower lip, for example in the closure phase of bilabial articulations such as [p], [m]. According to some investigations (Öhman *et al.*, 1965, p. 9) the levator anguli oris and its antagonist the depressor labii inferior function in achieving a graded upward movement of the lower lip.

### b. Zygomaticus Major

The zygomaticus major has already been discussed in Section IV.B.6.*b*. As the fibres travel slightly downward towards the angles of the mouth the muscle can draw the angles upwards as well as laterally. This action is probably important during articulation of [f].

## 8. Muscles that Lower the Angles of the Mouth

### a. Depressor Anguli Oris

*General description:* This muscle is also known as the triangularis because of its flat triangular shape.
*Origin:* Front surface of the mandible slightly lateral to the mid-line (Fig. 32).
*Course:* Vertically upwards.
*Insertion:* Most fibres insert into the orbicularis oris at the angles of the mouth.
*Innervation:* Facial (seventh cranial) nerve.
*Function:* The main function of the muscle is to depress the angles of the mouth. The muscle probably also acts synergistically to the depressor labii inferior in lowering the lower lip for the release of bilabial stops. An additional function of the muscle during the production of close vowels such as [i], [e] with a high mandible position, has been suggested by some investigations (Öhman *et al.*, 1965, p. 7). It is claimed that protagonist activity in this muscle may be necessary to prevent the lips closing off the mouth orifice during these vowels.

## b. Platysma

*General description:* The platysma muscle consists of a thin, quadrilateral sheet of fibres situated on the side of the neck and chin.
*Origin:* Upper pectoral and deltoid regions.
*Course:* Upwards and forwards towards the mandible.
*Insertion:* Partly into lower border of the mandible, interdigitating with the depressor labii inferior and depressor anguli oris. The anterior fibres sweep towards the median line where they decussate with fibres from the other side on the surface of the chin.
*Innervation:* Facial (seventh cranial) nerve.
*Function:* The muscle can have some effect as a synergist to the depressor anguli oris and the depressor labii inferior in drawing down the angles of the mouth. At the same time the muscle probably acts synergistically to the mentalis and orbicularis oris in protruding the lips for close rounded vowels such as [u], [y].

# V. The Physiology of the Velum

## A. General Description of the Velum

The velum or soft palate, can be regarded as a flexible extension of the hard palate (see above Fig. 22). It takes the form of a thin sheet consisting mainly of muscle fibres, tissue, blood vessels, nerves, and glands, which function to separate the nasal from the oral cavities. When lowered, air is able to pass into both the oral and nasal cavities; this happens for instance during the production of nasal articulations such as [m], [n] etc. When fully raised, the velum seals off the nasal cavity and air is directed out of the oral cavity only. It should be noted here that the nasal seal is frequently not complete during the production of many oral sounds in English; in many speakers' articulation of vowels, for example, some air flow out of the nose can be detected. The raised configuration occurs during normal oral articulations such as [t], [d], [p] etc. It has been suggested that there are only two modes of activity of the velum at the muscular level, the raising and lowering, and that any intermediate positions the velum might assume during speech production would be the result of biomechanical constraints of the articulatory mechanisms and differences in the timing with which the two modes are applied (Moll and Shriner, 1967, p. 68). This theory should be regarded with caution, however, as it seems possible that the velum is indeed capable of delicate muscular control necessary for achieving a critical ratio of areas of opening between the nasal and oral cavities.

The velum has three main attachments. Anteriorly, it is attached to the hard palate. Superiorly, it is fixed to the skull by two sets of muscles, whose fibres run down the sides of the nasal cavity into the lateral margins of the velum. Inferiorly, the velum is attached to the tongue and the pharynx. Muscle fibres inserting into the velum from these three attachments permit the main raising and lowering movements.

A small muscular flap, the uvula, is attached to the posterior edge of the velum. Its role is probably not so important in speech production except perhaps as an active articulator in the trilled uvular [R] and as a passive articulator during post-velar consonants such as [χ].

## B. The Muscles of the Velum

The muscles of the velum and their main functions are as follows:

1. Elevators:            *a*. levator palatini
                         *b*. musculus uvulae

2. Tensor:               *a*. tensor palatini
3. Depressors:           *a*. palatoglossus
                         *b*. palatopharyngeus

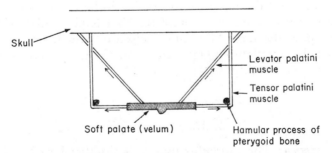

Fig. 33 The horizontal stretching action of the tensor palatini and the elevating action of the levator palatini. (After Van Riper and Irwin, 1958.)

The functions of the most important of these muscles are illustrated schematically in Fig. 33.

## 1. Muscles that Elevate the Velum

### a. Levator Palatini

*General description:* The levator palatini is the largest and strongest of the velic muscles.

*Origin:* Petrous part of the temporal bone of the skull.

*Course:* The fibres course downwards and forwards along the superior lateral pharyngeal wall. The fibres converge slightly near their insertion.

*Insertion:* The posterior surface of the velum, most muscle fibres interdigitating with their fellows from the other side.

*Innervation:* The vagus (tenth cranial) and facial (seventh cranial) nerves.

*Function:* The protagonist activity of the levator palatini is to elevate the velum upwards and posteriorly during the production of non-nasal articulations. Various electromyographic and cinefluorographic studies (Lubker, 1968; Fritzell, 1969) have shown a clear relationship between the raising movement of the velum and electrical activity in this muscle. The activity was normally found to be greater for stop articulations than for vowels (Calnan, 1953; Bell-Berti, 1973).

Activity of the levator muscle is probably accompanied by synergistic contraction of the tensor palatini which serves to stretch the velum sideways as shown in Fig. 33 (Van Riper and Irwin, 1958, p. 389). The amount of this synergistic activity, however, seems to vary considerably from subject to subject (Fritzell, 1969).

It is possible that simultaneous contraction of the constrictor pharyngis superior (see Section VI.B) takes place with the levator in helping to close off the nasal cavity. It should be noted, however, that this closure is very often not complete. Van Riper and Irwin (1958, p. 393) employ the term "functional closure" which means that the closure is only complete enough "to avoid the direct auditory consequencies of open nasality."

### b. Musculus Uvulae

*General description:* The musculus uvulae is situated largely within the uvula which protudes from the posterior, free end of the velum.

*Origin:* The posterior nasal spine and palatine aponeurosis, which forms the attachment of the velum to the posterior part of the hard palate.

*Course:* Medially from both sides between the layers of the palatopharyngeus (see below).

*Insertion:* The fibres interdigitate with each other before insertion into the mucous membrane of the uvula.

*Innervation:* Spinal accessory nerve, through the pharyngeal plexus.

*Function:* The primary function of this muscle is to shorten the uvula bringing the structure upwards and backwards.

It thus acts synergistically to the levator palatini and the pharyngeal muscles in closing off the nasopharynx from the oropharynx. The muscle also probably plays some role in setting the uvula position for the articulation of the trilled uvular [R].

## 2. Muscles that Tense the Velum

### a. Tensor Palatini

*General description:* The tensor palatini is a triangular shaped muscle situated anterior and lateral to the levator palatini.

*Origin:* The base of the medial pterygoid plate on the inferior surface of the sphenoid bone of the skull and the lateral wall of the Eustachian tube (Cunningham, 1972, pp. 292–295).

*Course:* Downwards and forwards along the medial pterygoid plate.

*Insertion:* The fibres insert into a tendon which passes around the hamulus of the medial pterygoid plate ending spread out along the palatal aponeurosis (Fig. 33).

*Innervation:* The mandibular division of the trigeminal (fifth cranial) nerve.

*Function:* The protagonist activity of this muscle is to spread out and tense the velum. This activity is said to take place simultaneous to the raising activity of the levator in closing off the velopharyngeal port, at least in some subjects. Figure 33 illustrates how this synergistic activity would take place. Other synergistic muscles to this closure activity would be the sphincter muscles of the pharynx (see Section VI.B) although, because of the relatively slow contraction time of these large pharyngeal sphincter muscles they probably cannot undergo rapid changes in tension during connected speech.

Some writers have suggested that contraction in the tensor muscle may be part of a "ready" activity for an utterance (Fritzell, 1969). This preparatory activity would include tensing of the velum by the tensor muscle, and slight elevation by the levator muscle. The detailed function of this muscle is a little unclear at present largely because of its relative inaccessibility to instrumental investigation (MacNeilage, 1972).

### 3. Muscles that Lower the Velum

#### a. Palatoglossus

The palatoglossus has already been discussed under muscles of the tongue (Section II) as one of the lingual elevators. When the tongue is fixed, however, the muscle will function to lower the velum for the production of nasal articulations. Because of the muscular linkage between the tongue and the velum provided by this muscle, the velum will be dragged down lower during the production of open vowels such as [a] and will be in a relatively higher position during production of close vowels such as [u] (Harrington, 1944; Moll, 1962; Moll and Shriner, 1967). This would explain the frequently noted observation that close vowels are less susceptible to nasality than open vowels.

It seems that the palatoglossus is the main antagonist muscle to the levator palatini in lowering the velum during speech, although electromyographic activity in this muscle has not always been observed to accompany nasalized sounds (Bell-Berti, 1972). It may be that in some subjects, a passive relaxation of the palatal muscles accompanies nasalization.

#### b. Palatopharyngeus

*General description:* A long, thin muscle which together with mucous membrane forms the posterior faucial pillars.
*Origin:* Most of the fibres arise in the velum, with many fibres interdigitating with those of the other side.
*Course:* The fibres course laterally and downward.
*Insertion:* The fibres insert with the stylopharyngeus muscle onto the posterior border of the thyroid cartilage and into the lateral pharyngeal wall.
*Innervation:* Vagus (tenth cranial) nerve.
*Function:* The protagonist activity of this muscle is to pull down on the velum, when acting from a fixed larynx and pharyngeal wall. The action is synergistic to the palatoglossus, and probably also the constrictor pharyngis superior, during the production of oral articulations.

When acting from a fixed velum, the palatopharyngeus can conceivably be regarded as an extrinsic muscle of the larynx raising the thyroid cartilage. This activity probably takes place during the first stage of swallowing. Also because of this attachment to the larynx, it is possible that larynx movement will affect the height of the velum (Moll and Shriner, 1967, p. 66; Podvinec, 1952).

## VI. Physiology of the Pharynx

### A. General Outline of the Pharynx

There is probably some point in considering the pharynx as an active articulator in the vocal tract as its diameter can be altered considerably during speech. As shown above, the anterior–posterior dimension of the pharynx can be altered by the position of the posterior part of the tongue, a fronted lingual articulation such as [i] resulting in a large anterior, posterior dimension, and retracted articulation such as [ɑ] resulting in a narrow dimension.

In addition, the anterior–posterior dimension of the pharynx in the region of the velum can also be altered by the movements of that organ.

The lateral dimension of the pharynx can also be varied, this time by the muscles of the pharynx itself, which have basically a sphincter function. Isotonic contraction of these sphincter muscles will narrow the pharynx and isometric contraction will serve to tense the wall of the pharynx. This latter activity will have considerable effect on the resonance quality of the laryngeal tone giving it a metallic, strident quality. This isometric tensing of the pharynx may be important during the production of the so-called tense articulations such as the initial Korean stop [t] in the word "ddæ" meaning "dirt" (Hardcastle, 1973).

Movements of the pharyngeal wall by means of the pharyngeal constrictor muscles will take place relatively slowly because of the size and shape of these muscles. This means that rapid fluctuations in the lateral width of the pharynx probably do not occur during speech production.

### B. Muscles of the Pharynx

There are three sphincter muscles of the pharynx which function to narrow the pharyngeal tube. They are the constrictor pharyngis superior, the constrictor pharyngis medius, and the constrictor pharyngis inferior (Cunningham, 1972, pp. 291, 292). In addition there are two muscles, the stylopharyngeus and salpingopharyngeus which function to draw up the walls of the pharynx, an action which is important during swallowing.

As the role of these muscles during speech articulation is uncertain, at present they will only be described briefly.

## a. Constrictor Pharyngis Superior

*General description:* This muscle is the most superiorly placed of the pharyngeal constrictors. It consists of a broad quadrilateral mass of fibres.

*Origin:* Several different origins including the lower border of the pterygoid plate and the hamular process, the pterygomandibular raphe, the posterior end of the mylohyoid line on the mandible and the sides of the tongue (scattered fibres only).

*Course:* Posteriorly, some fibres travelling slightly upwards. Many fibres interdigitate with the palatopharyngeus muscle.

*Insertion:* The fibres interdigitate posteriorly with their fellows from the other side.

*Innervation:* Vagus (tenth cranial) nerve.

*Function:* The protagonist activity of the muscle is a sphincter function narrowing the upper walls of the pharynx. Together with some fibres of the palatopharyngeus muscle, contraction of the superior constrictor in some speakers forms a bulge of muscular tissue called Passavant's cushion situated in a direct line posterior to the hard palate. This activity probably aids the levator and tensor palatini in closing off the velopharyngeal valve during the production of non-nasal articulations.

## b. Constrictor Pharyngis Medius

This muscle has already been described under the suprahyoid musculature (Chapter 4, Section III.A.1), as one of the muscles which move the hyoid bone. When the hyoid is fixed, however, the muscle can act to narrow the pharynx by the sphincter activity. Activity of the muscle probably takes place during the articulation of sounds made in the posterior part of the oral region such as [k], [u] etc.

## c. Constrictor Pharyngis Inferior

*General description:* The broadest and thickest of the constrictor muscles.

*Origin:* Cricoid and thyroid cartilages (along the whole extent of the oblique line).

*Course:* The fibres diverge greatly as they travel posteriorly and medialward. The superior fibres rise obliquely decussating with a large part of the medial constrictor.

*Insertion:* Most of the fibres interdigitate with their fellows from the other side into the posterior pharyngeal raphe. Some of the inferior fibres (sometimes called the cricopharyngeus muscle) form a sphincter around the esophagus. Contraction of these inferior fibres are especially important in setting the aperture of the esophagus for "esophageal" speech.

*Innervation:* The vagus (tenth cranial) nerve, particularly the external laryngeal branch.

*Function:* From a fixed larynx the muscle can contract to constrict the lower part of the pharynx thus narrowing it by a sphincter action. This activity is especially important during swallowing.

### d. *Stylopharyngeus* and e. *Salpingopharyngeus*

These muscles will not be described in detail as it is uncertain whether they play any active role in speech production. They may act synergistically to other pharyngeal and palatal muscles in helping to close off the velopharyngeal port. The stylopharyngeus can also raise the larynx so can be regarded as one of the extrinsic laryngeal muscles.

# 6

# Concluding Remarks: Approaches to a Physiological Theory of Phonetics

## I. The Place of Physiology in Phonetic Theory

It has already been indicated earlier that one of the most important aims of current phonetic research is to describe accurately the various articulatory events that take place during speech production. Such a description should include not only the positions and movements of various muscles involved in the speech production process but also the co-ordination, both temporal and spatial, of these muscular activities by neurological functions. With a framework of the anatomical and physiological structure of the oral system such as outlined in the previous chapters, one can proceed to synthesize this information and to begin to suggest more adequate physiological correlations of basic articulatory parameters. In this context "articulation" at the phonetic level refers to the changing surface configurations of the vocal tract, while "physiology" refers to the means by which these changes are achieved.

It is proposed in this concluding chapter to indicate the direction that attempts to formulate a complete physiological theory of phonetics should take.

## II. Some Correlations between Physiological Mechanisms and Basic Articulatory Categories

To a certain extent it is already possible, in a gross way, to specify some physiological aspects of phonetic theory. Some basic articulatory categories, for example, can be correlated with specific groups of lingual muscles or specific muscular activity. Some such categories will be discussed briefly below.

### A. Vocoid and Contoid

In Chapter 5 it was seen how the muscles of the tongue can be conveniently divided into an extrinsic and an intrinsic group. The extrinsic group, consisting of the genioglossus, styloglossus, hyoglossus and palatoglossus muscles have their origins outside the tongue and are mainly responsible for altering the gross position of the body of the tongue in the mouth. The intrinsic muscles, on the other hand, comprising the longitudinalis superior and inferior, the verticalis, and the transversus are located entirely within the body of the tongue and so are responsible for the most part for altering the shape of the tongue only.

The two muscle groups differ anatomically as well as functionally. In general, the extrinsic muscles are larger, slower, capable of exerting greater tension. The intrinsic muscles, by contrast, are smaller, faster, lighter, and usually are relatively incapable of exerting great tension (Perkell, 1969, p. 61). The intrinsic muscles also probably have much lower innervation ratios (see Chapter 1, Section II.D.3) of the motor units innervating them than the extrinsic muscles. This means the intrinsic muscles are capable of producing a wide variety of delicately controlled lingual shapes, whereas the extrinsic muscles are capable mainly of achieving gross differences only in the position of the tongue.

The two muscle systems can be correlated to a certain extent with two of the most basic phonetic categories—vocoids and contoids (henceforth V and C). These terms are used by Pike (1943, p. 78). The articulation of vocoids primarily involves gross positioning of the tongue body irrespective of any delicate adjustments of the surface configuration: the extrinsic system, therefore, is probably mainly responsible with the intrinsic system playing a minor role only. Contoids, on the other hand, require not only positioning of the tongue body at certain points in the oral region, but also often extremely delicate adjustments of the surface configuration. Contoid articulation thus probably utilizes maximally both the extrinsic system for the gross movements, and the intrinsic system for the delicate shape adjustments.

The possible interaction of the extrinsic and intrinsic systems in the production of vocoids and contoids generates some interesting hypotheses regarding coarticulation phonema. The interaction of the extrinsic and intrinsic muscle groups can help to explain, for instance, coarticulation features in a VCV-type sequence. Here the contoid articulation can be regarded as a gesture superimposed on a basically diphthongal, extrinsically-achieved V–V gesture (Öhman, 1966, p. 166; Perkell, 1969, pp. 61–62).

The intrinsic system, responsible for any delicately controlled tongue configuration required for the contoid, may be regarded as acting largely independently of the slower, continuously-varying vocoid-producing system. Thus in a sequence such as [a s i] the particular tongue configuration for the [s], involving among other things the production of a central groove by the intrinsic musculature is probably beginning to be formed during the articulation of [a].

## B. Stop and Fricative

Different manner categories of contoid articulation can also be described in physiological terms. The categories stop and fricative for example can be differentiated with reference to the type of muscular activity employed in their articulation. For the production of a stop, a ballistic type muscular contraction (see Chapter 2, Section III.B) is necessary, i.e. one involving primarily protagonist muscles acting relatively independently of antagonist muscles. Thus a ballistic activity of the longitudinalis superior brings the tip of the tongue upwards to make contact with the alveolar ridge during articulation of the stop [t] in a sequence such as [i t i]. In the articulation of [k] the velar contact is made primarily by ballistic contraction of the longitudinalis inferior muscle. Of course for the production of both these stops there can be synergistic activity from other muscles as well.

A fricative, on the other hand, requires a far more delicate balance of protagonist and antagonist muscles to create the specific stricture required to maintain the turbulent flow of air necessary for its production. In general terms then, fricatives can be said to require more delicate neuromuscular control than stops. One of the possible effects of this greater precision is that the articulators involved in the production of a fricative might move more slowly than for the production of a stop. MacNeilage (1972, p. 27) has suggested this as one of the possible explanations for the frequently observed lengthening of vowels before fricatives (Lehiste, 1970).

## C. Stop and Tap

The physiological parameter of rate of muscular contraction (see Chapter 2) may be used to distinguish between stops and taps. As with a stop, tap articulation requires gross positioning of the tongue body by the extrinsic system and a rapid ballistic-type muscular contraction such that one articulator is "thrown against" another. In this respect it is similar to the ballistic movement of a stop. A major difference, however, lies in the rate of movement; the tap being very much faster. There may also be aerodynamic factors involved, caused by the speed of articulation, which do not apply to a stop. It is interesting to note that most taps occur in the dental and alveolar regions (Ladefoged, 1971, p. 50). The muscles of the tongue tip–blade system (Chapter 5, Section II.C) that are primarily responsible for tap articulation (i.e. longitudinalis superior and verticalis) are probably particularly suitable for undergoing the rapid contractions necessary for tap articulation. One of the reasons for this is probably that these intrinsic muscles are in general lighter and smaller than other tongue muscles and so in general may contract faster (Cunningham, 1964, p. 268). This is perhaps why the production of taps usually occurs in the front part of the mouth with apical articulation.

## D. Flap Articulation

Flap articulation is different from a tap in that it usually involves retroflexion of the tip and a forward movement striking or flapping against the alveolar ridge as it passes (Abercrombie, 1967, pp. 49–50). The movement is essentially an apical movement, and in this respect it is similar to a tap. Both movements probably employ similar extrinsic and intrinsic muscles, the longitudinalis superior being the protagonist muscle for the retroflexion movement, and the longitudinalis inferior and anterior part of the genioglossus for the forward flapping movement. The degree of tension exerted by the longitudinalis superior in the flap, however, is probably greater than in the tap. The greater degree of contraction produces an upward–backward movement of the tip and blade essential for retroflexion; an upward movement only is sufficient for tap articulation.

## E. Trill Articulation

In the articulation of an alveolar trill, the tongue tip is held, by
balanced contraction of protagonist and antagonist muscles of the
intrinsic and extrinsic group, lightly against the alveolar ridge, and set
in vibration by the airstream passing out through the oral cavity. The
control necessary to place the tip in the correct position probably
comes primarily from the longitudinalis superior muscle with the
anterior genioglossus and the longitudinalis inferior acting as antagonists.
The rate of vibration of the tip against the alveolar ridge, contingent
upon such factors as tension of the muscles, velocity of air-flow, closeness
of constriction etc. can be quite high, up to as much as 30 Hz (Stetson,
1951). The physiological mechanisms involved in trill articulation are
thus quite different from tap or flap articulation although they can
all be produced in roughly the same area of the mouth using the same
articulatory organs. The degree of controlled muscular contraction,
i.e. the degree of interaction between protagonist and antagonist muscles
necessary for trills is similar to that used by fricatives, so there is probably
some justification in regarding a trill as physiologically more similar
to fricative articulations than to tap or flap articulation.

## F. Problems Involved in Formulating Relationships Between Particular Physical Mechanisms and Articulatory Manner Categories

Thus it is possible, as is shown above, at a simplistic level to specify
some basic articulatory manner categories in terms of physiological
mechanisms underlying them. For example, one can posit a general
relationship between the contributions of different muscular systems
of the tongue and the basic division of sounds into vocoids and contoids
(see Section II.A); vocoids using principally the extrinsic muscle
system and contoids both the extrinsic and intrinsic systems. However,
between different contoid articulations, the involvement of extrinsic
and intrinsic systems may vary considerably. Thus, within the manner
category stop (Section II.B), articulations involving the back part of the
tongue, e.g. velar stops, may adopt very different tongue postures from
alveolar articulations; one can probably even go so far as to say velar
stop articulations make more use of extrinsic muscles (e.g. styloglossus
and palatoglossus) than do alveolar stop articulations, where the

particular tongue configuration required relies to a larger extent on intrinsic muscles such as the longitudinalis superior and the verticalis to form the necessary closure with the tip and blade.

Another difficulty arises when one attempts to posit different physiological mechanisms for different manner categories such as those mentioned above. What are often regarded as two different manner categories may rely on rather similar physiological mechanisms for their articulation. Thus as was seen in Section II.E, trill articulation may be more similar physiologically to fricative articulation than to tap or flap articulation.

As our knowledge of the physiology of the oral region becomes more complete, it will become easier to posit one-to-one relationships between articulatory parameters and physiological mechanisms. If then a particular manner category has no one-to-one relationship with some physiological mechanism it would perhaps have to be revised. Various recent attempts (Peterson and Shoup, 1966; Ladefoged, 1971) to specify more closely the physiological mechanisms of speech have been promising, but much more detailed research is necessary before we can confidently specify any one-to-one relationship between articulatory and physiological activities. A start has been made, however, in Chapter 5, Section II.C by attempting to provide detailed physiological correlates for different lingual parameters. In that section the different tongue shapes and motions used in speech production were specified in terms of the interaction of seven articulatory parameters. An attempt was also made on a speculative basis to specify the lingual physiological mechanisms underlying each of these articulatory parameters. To achieve a really comprehensive theory of linguistic performance at the phonetic level, it should be possible to allocate quantitative values not only to the articulatory parameters of a given articulation, but also to the individual contributions of the muscles and muscle systems participating in the articulation. Thanks to various instrumental techniques, we can begin to quantify the parametric articulatory values of speech events, but reliable quantification of the muscular contributions is a very long way ahead at the moment, given the current relative inefficiency of such techniques as electromyography. What we can do at the moment is to attempt better quantification of articulatory parameters with the help of techniques such as cinefluorography and electropalatography, and if not quantify the muscular contributions at least try to identify theoretically, the muscles involved in particular articulations. As an example of this approach to the fringes of a physiological theory of phonetics, it may be interesting to look in detail, as an example, at the articulation of the voiceless grooved alveolar fricative [s], and speculate about its articulatory and physiological make-up. Attention will be focused primarily on the lingual articulation of this fricative.


# III. Articulation of the Complex Fricative [s]


The grooved fricative [s] has frequently been described as a "complex" articulation requiring maximum delicacy both of muscular control and sensory feedback for its production (Peterson and Shoup, 1966). Just what "complexity" means in terms of physiological mechanisms can be illustrated by a detailed description of this articulation in terms of the seven lingual parameters described in Chapter 5, Section II.C.

The production of [s] in the environment [ə s ə] is considered. Three phases of the articulation are described—an approach to the target position for [s], a hold phase where a specific tongue configuration is maintained during the production of the turbulence in the airstream, and the release phase where the tongue returns to the [ə] position.


## A. The Approach Phase

From the position for [ə], the whole tongue body moves forward and upwards towards the alveolar region (parameters 1 and 2) by the combined effort of the posterior part of the genioglossus, the styloglossus and palatoglossus. As the tongue moves forward, a concave configuration forms in the body of the tongue due mainly to contraction of the styloglossus and palatoglossus (parameter 5). At the same time also, the tip–blade system is beginning to form a central groove (parameter 6) by contraction mainly of the median part of the verticalis and the superficial transversus fibres. Simultaneously with the forward movement of the tongue body, the mandible moves slightly forward and upwards. The mandibular elevators including the temporalis, masseter, pterygoideus internus, and possibly also the pterygoideus externus (see Chapter 5, Section III.B) are mainly responsible for this movement. The lips also are beginning to move into a spread position under the influence of contraction of the buccinator, zygomaticus major and the risorius muscles (see Chapter 5, Section IV.B).

## B. The Hold Phase

The specific lingual configuration of [s], involving the formation of a central groove in the tip–blade tongue system while the sides of the tongue are held firmly between the lateral dentition is extremely complex and requires the concerted activity of many muscular systems. The central groove in the tip–blade itself (parameter 6) is controlled primarily by balanced contraction of both extrinsic and intrinsic lingual muscles. The protagonist muscles are probably the median verticalis and superior part of the transversus, with the longitudinalis inferior acting synergistically to lower the central part of the tip. Contraction of the verticalis muscle and the posterior part of the genioglossus probably contribute to the formation of a lateral seal between the upper and lower lateral teeth thus preventing air from escaping there. To achieve this lateral seal, spreading of the blade is necessary (parameter 7). Balanced contraction by the longitudinalis superior and the anterior part of the genioglossus ensures that the tip is lowered to just the right degree to allow the airstream to pass out of the central groove (parameter 6).

At the same time as the central groove is being maintained, the whole tongue body is held forward in the mouth, chiefly by the protagonist activity of the posterior genioglossus (parameter 1). The anterior suprahyoid muscles probably act synergistically in this movement, the mandible meanwhile being held in an appropriate position by the elevator muscles. To prevent the tongue moving forward too far in the mouth, the depressors of the tongue, the hyoglossus and the infrahyoid musculature probably contract antagonistically.

It was mentioned above that the styloglossus and palatoglossus (acting from a fixed velum) contribute to the forward upward movement of the tongue body, and because these muscles are inserted along the lateral margins of the tongue the back part forms a concave or sulcalized configuration (parameter 5). This configuration may be important for achieving the specific acoustic characteristics associated with normal articulation of this sound.

Articulation of [s] depends probably to a large extent on the precise control of the anterior central groove. Just the right amount of balanced tension must be exerted by the longitudinalis superior and the anterior genioglossus (with the longitudinalis inferior acting synergistically) to lower the central part of the tip sufficiently to allow the air to pass. There is thus a mutual dependency of air-flow, orifice size, and pressure ratio (Warren and Du Bois, 1964). This sustained balanced contraction is necessary throughout the critical hold phase.

## C. The Release Phase

Both the body and tip–blade systems are lowered and slightly retracted mainly by the hyoglossus and inferior infrahyoids (parameters 1 to 4) for the release. The mandible is lowered by the anterior suprahyoid musculature.

## D. The Fricative [s] as a "Complex" Articulation

We can see from the above description that [s] makes use of all seven lingual parameters. What makes the articulation particularly complex, however, is that not only are all the parameters utilized at some stage in the articulation, but very delicate control takes place for each parameter.

Not all articulations utilize these parameters to the same extent as [s]. Thus most vocoids, for example, probably only involve parameters 1, 2, and possibly 3, 4, and 5. It can be said then that, in a sense, some articulations are more complex than others, with "complexity" being defined both in terms of the number of articulatory parameters active and the delicacy of control exerted on those parameters by their underlying physiological mechanisms. In general, complex articulations would involve a greater number of the seven articulatory parameters than less complex articulations; however, each parameter probably does not require the same degree of physiological control. Thus, for example, parameters 1 and 2, involving gross movement of the tongue body probably do not employ such delicately controlled physiological mechanisms as degrees of central grooving of the tip–blade system (parameter 6). It may perhaps be possible to weight different parameters according to their place in a hierarchy of degrees of physiological delicacy required for their production. To a certain extent this is already possible by regarding those parameters primarily involved in activity of the extrinsic muscle system of the tongue as being less complex than those requiring contribution from both the extrinsic and intrinsic systems.

We could conceivably proceed along similar lines in specifying articulatory parameters for the other speech organs in the oral region such as the lips, mandible and velum. The problem would then be to compare the contribution of these parameters to those of the tongue. The fricative [f], for example, involving probably maximal utilization of all labial articulatory parameters and minimal utilization of lingual parameters may perhaps be rightly regarded as equivalent in complexity to the grooved fricative [s].

Adopting a parametric approach such as that outlined above, we can, at least in theory, perhaps arrange all sounds in a cline from simple to complex articulations; the complex exhibiting maximally delicate interrelationships between both the articulatory parameters and physiological mechanisms.

This concept of complexity may have applications throughout nearly all sciences involved with speech. For example, a parametric approach specifying not only precisely defined articulatory parameters but also physiological mechanisms underlying them may be more suitable as a unifying theory behind speech acquisition. It is possible that children, in acquiring speech, progress from simple to complex articulations, i.e. they acquire more and more interrelationships between different parameters. (Studies by Templin (1957), Poole (1934) and Jakobson (1944) have shown that children normally acquire fricatives [s], [ʃ] later than [p], [m], [d].) This sort of parametric approach also may be more applicable in explaining certain aspects of historical sound change; it may be possible, for instance, to posit a general tendency in a given language for sounds to change throughout time from more complex to more simple articulations.

Studies of slips of the tongue in English support the hypothesis that some articulations particularly the so-called grooved fricatives [s] and [ʃ] are more complex than other sounds. It has been noted for instance that these fricatives are more likely to interact in tongue slips particularly as regards place of articulation than hypothetically less complex articulations such as plosives and other consonant categories (Boomer and Laver, 1968). This is reflected further in the maximal difficulty of tongue twisters involving alternations of voiceless fricatives [s] and [ʃ], e.g. "She sells sea-shells on the sea-shore", and the fact that the articulation of grooved fricatives usually poses severe difficulty for pathological patients with most types of sensori-motor impairments (Luchsinger and Arnold, 1970, p. 293).


# IV. Conclusion


To sum up, this chapter has been an attempt to indicate the direction which the formation of a comprehensive phonetic theory should take. Rather than specify in a general fashion, as is the practice in conventional phonetic theory, articulatory parameters such as place and manner of articulations such as [s], an attempt has been made here to specify not only the intersection of detailed articulatory parameters, but also to indicate the physiological mechanisms underlying these parameters by drawing on some of the material outlined in the preceding chapters.

An attempt has been made to indicate how one might utilize this approach in formulating an adequate objective definition of articulatory complexity.

It is hoped that the material contained in this book will have provided the reader with a basic background knowledge of the functioning of the speech mechanism and have opened up some possible new avenues of research. It is clear that a great deal of work still has to be done by researchers in many different disciplines including anatomy, physiology, neurology, linguistics, phonetics, speech pathology and psychology before we are in a position to offer a comprehensive account of the phonetic basis of linguistic performance. This book has attempted to provide at least part of the necessary theoretical framework for these researchers.

# References

Abd-el-Malek, S. (1939). Observations on the morphology of the human tongue, *Journal of Anatomy* **73**, 201–212.

Abercrombie, D. (1967). "Elements of General Phonetics" Edinburgh: Edinburgh University Press.

Adatia, A. K. and Gehring, E. N. (1971). Proprioceptive innervation of the tongue, *Journal of Anatomy* **110**, 215–220.

Andrew, B. L. (Ed.) (1966). "Control and Innervation of Skeletal Muscle" Edinburgh: E. and S. Livingstone.

Arnold, G. E. (1961). Physiology and pathology of the cricothyroid muscle, *Laryngoscope* **71**, 687–753.

Arnold, M. (1968). "Reconstructive Anatomy" Philadelphia: W. B. Saunders.

Barker, D. (Ed.) (1962). "Symposium on Muscle Receptors" Hong Kong: Hong Kong University Press.

Barron, D. H. (1936). A note on the course of the proprioceptive fibres from the tongue, *Anatomical Record* **66**, 11–15.

Békésy, G. von (1967), "Sensory Inhibition" Princeton: Princeton University Press.

Bell-Berti, F. (1973). "The Velopharyngeal Mechanism: An Electromyographic Study." Status Report on Speech Research (supplement) New York: Haskins Laboratories.

Bernstein, N. (1967). "The Co-ordination and Regulation of Movements" London, New York: Pergamon Press.

Bessou, P., Emonet-Dénand, F. and Laporte, Y. (1963). Relation entre la vitesse de conduction de fibres nerveuses motrices et le temps de contraction de leur unités motrices, *Comptes-Rendues de l'Académie de Sciences* **256**, 5625–5638.

Bessou, P., Emonet-Dénand, F. and Laporte, Y. (1965). Motor fibres innervating extrafusal and intrafusal muscle fibres in the cat, *Journal of Physiology* **180**, 649–672.

Boomer, D. S. and Laver, J. D. M. (1968). Slips of the tongue, *British Journal of Disorders of Communication* **3**, 1–11.

Bosma, J. F. (Ed.) (1967). "Symposium on Oral Sensation and Perception" Springfield, Illinois: Charles C. Thomas.

Bourne, G. H. (Ed.) (1972). "The Structure and Function of Muscle" 2nd edn. Vols 1 and 2 London, New York: Academic Press.

Bowman, J. P. (1971). "The Muscle Spindle and Neural Control of the Tongue" Springfield, Illinois: Charles C. Thomas.

Boyd, I. A. (1962). The structure and innervation of the nuclear-bag muscle fibre system and the nuclear-chain muscle fibre system in mammalian muscle spindles, *Philosophical Transactions of the Royal Society* (Series B) **245**, 81–136.

Boyd, I. A. and Davey, M. R. (1966). The composition of peripheral nerves, *In* "Control and Innervation of Sketetal Muscle" (Ed. B. L. Andrew) pp. 35–53. Edinburgh: E. and S. Livingstone.

Broad, D. J. (1973). Phonation, *In* "Normal Aspects of Speech, Hearing, and Language" (Ed. F. D. Minifie, T. J. Hixon and F. Williams) pp. 127–169 New Jersey: Prentice-Hall.

Buller, A. J. (1969). The physiology of the motor unit, *In* "Disorders of Voluntary Muscle" 2nd edn (Ed. J. N. Walton) pp. 17–27 London: J. and A. Churchill.

Calnan, J. (1953). Movements of the soft palate, *British Journal of Plastic Surgery* **5**, 280–296.

Campbell, E. J. (1958). "The Respiratory Muscles and the Mechanics of Breathing" London: Lloyd-Luke.

Chusid, J. G. and McDonald, J. J. (1967). "Correlative Neuroanatomy and Functional Neurology" Los Altos, California: Lange Medical Publishers.

Clough, J. F. M., Kernell, D. and Philipps, C. G. (1968). The distribution of monosynaptic excitation from the pyramidal tract and from primary spindle afferents to motoneurons of the baboon's hand and forearm, *Journal of Physiology* **198**, 145–166.

Cooper, S. (1953). Muscle spindles in the intrinsic muscles of the human tongue, *Journal of Physiology* **122**, 193–202.

Cooper, S. (1960). Muscle spindles and other muscle receptors, *In* "Structure and Function of Muscle" (Ed. G. H. Bourne) Vol. 1, pp. 381–420 New York, London: Academic Press.

Craik, K. J. W. (1947). Theory of the human operator in control systems. 1. The operator as an engineering system, *British Journal of Psychology* **38**, 56–61.

Cunningham, D. J. (1964). "Cunningham's Textbook of Anatomy" 10th edn (Ed. G. J. Romanes) London: Oxford University Press.

Cunningham, D. J. (1972). "Cunningham's Textbook of Anatomy" 11th edn (Ed. G. J. Romanes) London: Oxford University Press.

Dabelow, R. (1951). Vorstudien zu einer Betrachtung der Zunge als funktionelles System: II Die Muskulatur und ihre bindegewebigen Insertionen (Fascia linguae und Septum), *Morphologisches Jahrbuch* **91**, 33–73.

Daniloff, R. G. and Hammarberg, R. E. (1973). On defining coarticulation, *Journal of Phonetics* **1**, 239–248.

Daniloff, R. and Moll, K. (1968). Co-articulation of lip rounding, *Journal of Speech and Hearing Research* **11**, 707–721.

Davson, H. (1970). "A Textbook of General Physiology" 4th edn London: J. and A. Churchill.

Diamond, M. (1952). "Dental Anatomy" 3rd edn New York: Macmillan.

Di Salvo, N. A. (1961). Neuromuscular mechanisms involved in mandibular movement and posture, *American Journal of Orthodontics* **47**, 330–342.

Dixon, A. D. (1962). The position, incidence and origin of sensory nerve terminations in oral mucous membrane, *Archives of Oral Biology* **7**, 39–48.

Draper, M. H., Ladefoged, P. and Whitteridge, D. (1959). Respiratory muscles in speech, *Journal of Speech and Hearing Research* **2**, 16–27.

Draper, M. H., Ladefoged, P. and Whitteridge, D. (1960). Expiratory pressures and air flow during speech, *British Medical Journal* **1**, 1837–1843.

Eccles, J. C. (1952), "The Neurophysiological Basis of Mind" Oxford: Oxford University Press.

Eccles, J. C. (1958). The physiology of imagination, *Scientific American* **65**, 1–11.

Eccles, J. C. (1973). "The Understanding of the Brain" New York: McGraw-Hill Co. Ltd.

Eccles, J. C., Ito, M. and Szentágothai, J. (1967), "The Cerebellum as a Neuronal Machine" Berlin: Springer.

Erlanger, J. and Gasser, H. S. (1937). "Electrical Signs of Nervous Activity" Philadelphia: University of Pennsylvania Press.

Faaborg-Andersen, K. (1965). "Electromyography of Laryngeal Muscles in Humans. Technics and Results" Basel: Karger.

Feneis, H. (1974). "Anatomisches Bildwörterbuch" 4th edn Stuttgart: Georg Thieme.

Fink, B. R. (1962). Tensor mechanism of the vocal folds, *Annals of Otology, Rhinology and Laryngology* **71,** 591–599.

Fritzell, B. (1969). The velopharyngeal muscles in speech: An electromyographic and cinefluorographic study, *Acta oto-laryngologica* Supplement 250.

Fromkin, V. A. (1966), Neuromuscular specification of linguistic units, *Language and Speech* **9,** 170–199.

Fry, D. B. (1957). Speech and language, *Journal of Laryngology and Otology* **71,** 434–452.

Fujimura, O. (1961). Bilabial stop and nasal consonants: a motion picture study and its acoustical implications, *Journal of Speech and Hearing Research* **4,** 233–247.

Fujimura, O. (1972). Acoustics of speech, *In* "Speech and Cortical Functioning" (Ed. J. H. Gilbert) pp. 107–167 New York, London: Academic Press.

Gammon, S. A., Smith, P. J., Daniloff, R. G. and Kim, C. W. (1971). Articulation and stress/juncture production under oral anesthetization and masking, *Journal of Speech and Hearing Research* **14,** 271–282.

Gelfan, S. (1955). Functional activity of muscle, *In* "A Textbook of Physiology" 17th edn (Ed. J. F. Fulton) pp. 123–158 Philadelphia: W. B. Saunders.

Gimson, A. C. (1970). "An Introduction to the Pronunciation of English" 2nd edn London: Edward Arnold.

Granit, R. (1966). "Proceedings of the First Nobel Symposium: Muscular Afferents and Motor Control" Stockholm: Almqvist and Wiksell.

Granit, R. (Ed.) (1970). "The Basis of Motor Control" New York, London: Academic Press.

Gray, J. A. B. (1959). Mechanical into electrical energy in certain mechanoreceptors, *Progress in Biophysics and Biophysical Chemistry* **9,** 285–324.

Grossman, R. C. (1964). Sensory innervation of the oral mucosa: a review, *Journal Southern California State Dental Association* **32,** 128–133.

Grossman, R. C. and Hattis, B. F. (1967). Oral mucosal sensory innervation and sensory experience: a review, *In* "Symposium on Oral Sensation and Perception" (Ed. J. F. Bosma) pp. 5–63 Springfield, Illinois: Charles C. Thomas.

Hardcastle, W. J. (1970). "The role of Tactile and Proprioceptive feedback in Speech Production", Work in Progress No. 4 pp. 100–112 Department of Linguistics, Edinburgh University.

Hardcastle, W. J. (1971). Electropalatography in the Investigation of Some Physiological Aspects of Speech Production Ph.D. Dissertation. Department of Linguistics, University of Edinburgh.

Hardcastle, W. J. (1973). Some observations on the tense-lax distinction in initial stops in Korean, *Journal of Phonetics* **1,** 263–272.

Hardcastle, W. J. (1974). Instrumental investigations of lingual activity during speech: a survey, *Phonetica* **29,** 129–157.

Hardcastle, W. J. (1975). Some aspects of speech production under controlled conditions of oral anaesthesia and auditory masking, *Journal of Phonetics* **3,** 197–214.

Harrington, R. (1944). A study of the mechanism of velopharyngeal closure, *Journal of Speech Disorders* **9**, 325–344.

Harris, K. S. (1974). Physiological aspects of articulatory behavior, *In* "Current Trends in Linguistics" (Ed. T. A. Sebeok) Vol. 12 The Hague: Mouton.

Harris, K. S., Lysaught, G. F. and Schvey, M. M. (1965). Some aspects of the production of oral and nasal labial stops, *Language and Speech* **8**, 135–147.

Head, H. and Holmes, G. (1920). "Studies in Neurology" London: Oxford Medical Publishers.

Henneman, E., Somjen, G. and Carpenter, D. O. (1965). Functional significance of cell size in spinal Motoneurons, *Journal of Neurophysiology* **28**, 560–580.

Hill, A. V. (1953). The mechanics of active muscle, *Proceedings of the Royal Society* (Series B) **141**, 104–117.

Hirano, M. and Smith, T. (1967). "Electromyographic study of Tongue Function in Speech: A Preliminary Report," Working Papers in Phonetics 7, pp. 46–56 University of California at Los Angeles.

Hirano, M., Ohala, J. and Vennard, W. (1969). The function of laryngeal muscles in regulating fundamental frequency and intensity of phonation, *Journal of Speech and Hearing Research* **12**, 616–628.

Hirose, H. and Gay, T. (1972). The activity of the intrinsic laryngeal muscles in voicing control, *Phonetica* **25**, 140–164.

Hixon, T. J. (1973). Respiratory function in speech, *In* "Normal Aspects of Speech, Hearing, and Language" (Ed. F. D. Minifie, T. J. Hixon and F. Williams) pp. 73–127 New Jersey: Prentice Hall.

Hixon, T. J., Klatt, D. and Mead, J. (1970). Influence of forced transglottal pressure changes on vocal fundamental frequency, Paper Read at Acoustical Society of America Meeting, Houston, Texas.

Hodgkin, A. L. (1964). "The Conduction of the Nervous Impulse" Sherrington Lectures No. 7 Liverpool: Liverpool University Press.

Hollien, H. (1962). Vocal fold thickness and fundamental frequency of phonation, *Journal of Speech and Hearing Research* **5**, 237–243.

Hollien, H. and Colton, R. H. (1969). Four laminagraphic studies of vocal fold thickness, *Folia Phoniatrica* **21**, 179–198.

Hollien, H. and Moore, G. P. (1960). Measurement of the vocal folds during changes in pitch, *Journal of Speech and Hearing Research* **3**, 157–165.

Hosokawa, H. (1961). Proprioceptive innervation of striated muscles in the territory of the cranial nerves, *Texas Reports on Biology and Medicine* **19**, 405–464.

Hudgins, C. V. and Stetson, R. H. (1937). Relative speed of articulatory movements, *Archives néerlandaises de phonétique expérimentale* **13**, 85–94.

Hursh, J. B. (1939). Conduction velocity and diameter of nerve fibres, *American Journal of Physiology* **127**, 131–139.

Huxley, H. E. (1965). The mechanism of muscular contraction, *Scientific American* **213**, 18–27.

Huxley, H. E. (1969). The mechanism of muscular contraction, *Science* **164**, 1356–1366.

Isshiki, N. (1959). Regulatory mechanism of the pitch and volume of voice, *Oto- rhino- and Laryngological Clinic, Kyoto* **52**, 1065–1094.

Jakobson, R. (1944). "Kindersprache, Aphasie und allgemeine Lautgesetze" Uppsala: Språkretenskapliga Sållskapets i Uppsala Förhandlingar.

Jansen, J. K. S. (1966). On fusimotor reflex activity, *In* "Proceedings of the First Nobel Symposium: Muscular Afferents and Motor Control" (Ed. R. Granit) Stockholm: Almqvist and Wiksell.

Jassem, W. and Morton, J. (1965). Acoustic correlates of stress, *Language and Speech* **8**, 159–179.

Judson, L. S. V. and Weaver, A. T. (1965). "Voice Science" 2nd edn New York: Appleton-Century-Crofts.

Kagaya, R. (1971). Laryngeal gestures in Korean stop consonants. "Annual Bulletin", Research Institute of Logopedics and Phoniatrics, University of Tokyo 5, pp. 15–23.

Kaiser, L. (1934). Some properties of the speech muscles and the influence thereof on language, *Archives néerlandaises de phonétique experimentale* **10**, 121–133.

Kamada, S. (1955). On the innervation especially sensory innervation of mucous membrane of the oral cavity of cat, *Archivum Histologicum Japonicum* **8**, 243–260.

Kantner, M. (1957). Neue morphologische Ergebnisse über die peripherischen Nerbenausbreitungen und ihre Deutung, *Acta Anatomica* (Basel) **31**, 397–425.

Kaplan, H. M. (1971). "Anatomy and Physiology of Speech" 2nd edn New York: McGraw-Hill Book Co. Ltd.

Katz, B. (1962). The transmission of impulses from nerve to muscle, and the sub-cellular unit of synaptic action, *Proceedings of the Royal Society* (Series B) **155**, 455–479.

Katz, B. (1966). "Nerve, Muscle and Synapse" New York: McGraw-Hill Book Co. Ltd.

Kawamura, Y., Majima, T. and Kato, I. (1967). Physiologic role of deep mechano-receptors in temporomandibular joint capsule, *Journal Osaka University Dental School* **7**, 63–76.

Kim, C. W. (1970). A theory of aspiration, *Phonetica* **21**, 107–116.

Klineberg, I., Greenfield, B. E. and Wyke, B. D. (1970). Afferent discharges from temporo-mandibular articular mechanoreceptors: an experimental study in the cat, *Archives of Oral Biology* **15**, 935–952.

Koepke, G. H. *et al.* (1958). Sequence of action of the diaphragm and intercostal muscles during respiration. I. inspiration, *Archives of Physical Medicine* **39**, 426–430.

Kuffler, S. W. and Hunt, C. C. (1952). The mammalian small nerve fibres; a system for efferent nervous regulation of muscle spindle discharge, *Research Publications. Association for Research in Nervous and Mental Diseases* **30**, 24–47.

Ladefoged, P. (1967). "Three Areas of Experimental Phonetics" London: Oxford University Press.

Ladefoged, P. (1971) "Preliminaries to Linguistic Phonetics" Chicago and London: University of Chicago Press.

Ladefoged, P. (1973). The features of the larynx, *Journal of Phonetics* **1**, 73–83.

Ladefoged, P., Draper, M. and Whitteridge, D. (1958). Syllables and stress, *Miscellanea Phonetica* **3**, 1–14.

Langworthy, O. R. (1924). Study of the innervation of the tongue musculature with particular reference to the proprioceptive mechanism, *Journal of Comparative Neurology* **36**, 273–293.

Lashley, K. S. (1951). The problem of serial order in behaviour, *In* "Cerebral Mechanisms in Behaviour" (Ed. L. A. Jeffress) New York: John Wiley and Sons.

Laver, J. (1969). "The Detection and Correction of Slips of the Tongue" Work in Progress No. 3, pp. 1–12 Department of Phonetics and Linguistics, Edinburgh University.

Lawson, W. A. and Bond, E. K. (1968). Speech and its relation to dentistry. II. The influence of oral structures on speech, *The Dental Practitioner* **19**, 113–118.

Lebrun, Y. (1966). Is stress essentially a thoracic or an abdominal pulse? A finding of not proven, *In* "Linguistic Research in Belgium" (Ed. Y. Lebrun) pp. 69–76 Welleren: Universa.

Lehiste, I. L. (1970). "Suprasegmentals" Cambridge, Mass.: MIT Press.

Leksell, L. (1945). The action potential and excitatory effects of the small ventral root fibres to skeletal muscle, *Acta Physiologica Scandinavica* **10** (Supplement 31).

Lenneberg, E. H. (1967). "Biological Foundations of Language" New York: John Wiley and Sons.

Liddell, E. G. T. and Sherrington, C. S. (1925). Recruitment and some other features of reflex inhibition, *Proceedings of the Royal Society* (Series B) **97**, 488—518.

Lieberman, P. (1960). Some acoustic correlates of word stress in American English, *Journal of the Acoustical Society of America* **32**, 451–454.

Lindblom, B. (1967). Vowel duration and a model of lip mandible coordination "Quarterly Progress and Status Report", Royal Institute of Technology, Stockholm 4, pp. 1–29.

Loewenstein, W. R. (1960). Biological transducers, *Scientific American* **203**, 98–108.

Lubker, J. F. (1968). An electromyographic-cinefluorographic investigation of velar function during normal speech articulation, *The Cleft Palate Journal* **5**, 1–18.

Luchsinger, R. and Arnold, G. F. (1970). "Handbuch der Stimm- und Sprachheilkunde" 3rd edn Wien: Springer.

Lullies, H. (1972). Stimme und Sprache, *In* Hören, Stimme, Gleichgewicht ("Physiology des Menschen", Vol. 12), Ed O. H. Gauer, K. Kramer and R. Jung.) pp. 215–258 München-Berlin-Wien: Urban and Schwarzenberg.

Luria, A. R. (1966). "Higher Cortical Functions in Man" New York: Basic Books.

MacNeilage, P. F. (1970). Motor control of serial ordering of speech, *Psychological Review* **77**, 182–196.

MacNeilage, P. F. (1972). Speech physiology, *In* "Speech and Cortical Functioning" (Ed. J. H. Gilbert) pp. 1–73 London, New York: Academic Press.

MacNeilage, P. F. and De Clerk, J. L. (1969). On the motor control of co-articulation in CVC monosyllables, *Journal of the Acoustical Society of America* **45**, 1217–1233.

MacNeilage, P. F. and Sholes, G. N. (1964). An electromyographic study of the tongue during vowel production, *Journal of Speech and Hearing Research* **7**, 209–232.

MacNeilage, P. F., Rootes, T. P. and Chase, R. A. (1967). Speech production and perception in a patient with severe impairment of somesthetic perception and motor control, *Journal of Speech and Hearing Research* **10**, 449–467.

Matthews, P. B. C. (1964) Muscle spindles and their motor control, *Physiological Review* **44**, 219–288.

Matthews, P. B. C. (1972). "Mammalian Muscle Receptors and Their Central Actions" London: Edward Arnold.

McCroskey, R. (1958). The relative contributions of auditory and tactile cues to certain aspects of speech, *Southern Speech Journal* **24**, 84–90.

McGlone, R. E. and Shipp, T. (1971). Some physiologic correlates of vocal-fry phonation, *Journal of Speech and Hearing Research* **14**, 769–775.

Merton, P. A. (1953). Speculations on the servo-control of movement, *In* "The Spinal Cord" (Ed. G. E. W. Wolstenholme) pp. 247–255 London: J. and A. Churchill.

Milner, P. M. (1967). "Physiological Psychology" Montreal: McGill University (mimeo).

Milner, P. H. (1970). "Physiological Psychology" London: Holt, Rinehart and Winston.

Miyawaki, K. (1974). A study of the musculature of the human tongue: observations on transport preparations of serial sections, "Annual Bulletin" Research Institute of Logopedics and Phoniatrics, University of Tokyo 8, pp. 23–50.

Moll, K. L. (1962). Velopharyngeal closure on vowels, *Journal of Speech and Hearing Research* **5**, 30–37.

Moll, K. L. and Shriner, T. H. (1967). Preliminary investigation of a new concept of velar activity during speech, *The Cleft Palate Journal* **4**, 58–69.

Öhman, S. E. G. (1966). Co-articulation in VCV utterances: spectrographic measurements, *Journal of the Acoustical Society of America* **39**, 151–168.

Öhman, S. E. G. (1967). Peripheral motor commands in labial articulation, "Quarterly Progress and Status Report", Royal Institute of Technology, Stockholm 4, pp. 30–63.

Öhman, S., Leanderson, R. and Persson, A. (1965). Electromyographic studies of facial muscles during speech, "Quarterly Progress and Status Report", Royal Institute of Technology, Stockholm 3, pp. 1–11.

Ormea, F. and Re, G. (1959). Strutture nervoze e funzione nervose della regione buccale, *Minerva dermatologica* **36**, 611–631.

Penfield, W. and Boldrey, E. (1937). Somatic motor and sensory representation in the cerebral cortex of man as studied by electrical stimulation, *Brain* **60**, 389–443.

Penfield, W. and Rasmussen, T. (1950). "The Cerebral Cortex of Man" New York: Macmillan.

Penfield, W. and Roberts, L. (1959). "Speech and Brain Mechanism" Princeton, N. J.: Princeton University Press.

Perkell, J. S. (1969). "Physiology of Speech Production: Results and Implications of a Quantitative Cineradiographic Study" Research Monograph No. 53 Cambridge, Mass., London: MIT Press.

Peterson, G. E. and Shoup, J. E. (1966). A physiological theory of phonetics, *Journal of Speech and Hearing Research* **9**, 5–67.

Pfaffmann, C. (1939). Afferent impulses from the teeth due to pressure and noxious stimulation, *Journal of Physiology* **97**, 207–219.

Pike, K. L. (1943). "Phonetics" Ann Arbor: University of Michigan Press.

Podvinec, S. (1952). The physiology and pathology of the soft palate, *Journal of Laryngology and Otology* **66**, 452–461.

Poole, J. (1934). Genetic development of articulation of consonant sounds in speech, *Elementary English Review* **11**, 159–161.

Ranson, S. W. and Clark, S. L. (1964). "The Anatomy of the Nervous System" Philadelphia, London: W. B. Saunders.

Rasch, P. J. and Burke, R. K. (1971). "Kinesiology and Applied Anatomy" 4th edn Philadelphia: Lea and Febiger.

Ringel, R. L. and Ewanowski, S. J. (1965). Oral perception: 1. Two-point discrimination, *Journal of Speech and Hearing Research* **8**, 389–398.

Ringel, R. L. and Steer, M. D. (1963). Some effects of tactile and auditory alterations on speech output, *Journal of Speech and Hearing Research* **6**, 369–378.

Roberts, T. D. M. (1966). "Basic Ideas in Neurophysiology" London: Butterworths.

Rossier, P. H., Buhlmann, A. A. and Wiesinger, K. (1960). "Respiration" St. Louis, Mo: C. V. Mosby Co.

Rushworth, G. (1969). Modification of gamma system activity in man, *In* "The Role of the Gamma System in Movement and Posture" (Ed. C. A. Swinyard) New York: Association for Aid of Crippled Children.

Saunders, W. H. (1964). "The Larynx" New Jersey: Ciba Pharmaceutical Company.

Sawashima, M. (1974). Laryngeal research in experimental phonetics, *In* "Current Trends in Linguistics" Vol. 12 (Ed. T. A. Sebeok) The Hague: Mouton.

Sawashima, M., Gay, T. and Harris, K. S. (1969). Laryngeal muscle activity during vocal pitch and intensity changes. Status Report on Speech Research 19/20, pp. 211–220 New York: Haskins Laboratories.

Schliesser, H. and Coleman, R. (1968). Effectiveness of certain procedures for alteration of auditory and oral tactile sensation for speech, *Perceptual and Motor Skills* **26**, 275–281.

Scott, C. M. and Ringel, R. L. (1971). Articulation without oral sensory control, *Journal of Speech and Hearing Research* **14**, 804–818.

Scott, J. H. and Symons, N. B. B. (1974). "Introduction to Dental Anatomy" 7th Edn Edinburgh: Churchill Livingstone.

Shipp, T. and McGlone, R. E. (1971). Laryngeal dynamics associated with voice frequency change, *Journal of Speech and Hearing Research* **14**, 761–768.

Shipp, T., McGlone, R. and Morrissey, P. (1972). Some physiologic correlates of voice frequency change, "Proceedings of the 7th International Congress of Phonetic Science" pp. 407–411 The Hague: Mouton.

Smith, T. and Hirano, M. (1968). "Experimental Investigations of the Muscular Control of the Tongue in Speech," Working Papers in Phonetics, Department of Linguistics, UCLA 10, pp. 145–156.

Sognnaes, R. F. (1954). Oral cavity, *In* "Histology" 1st edn (Ed. R. O. Greep) pp. 458–511 New York: Blakiston Co.

Sonesson, B. (1959). Die funktionelle Anatomie des Cricoarytenoidgelenkes, *Zeitschrift für Anatomie und Entwicklungsgeschichte* **121**, 292–303.

Sonesson, B. (1970). The functional anatomy of the speech organs, *In* "Manual of Phonetics" (Ed. B. Malmberg) pp. 45–75 Amsterdam: North Holland-Publishing Company.

Starling, E. H. (1941). "Principles of Human Physiology" 8th edn (Ed. C. Lovatt Evans) London: J. and A. Churchill.

Stetson, R. H. (1951). "Motor Phonetics" 2nd edn Amsterdam: North Holland-Publishing Company.

Stevens, K. N. and House, A. S. (1963). Perturbations of vowel articulations by consonantal context; an acoustical study, *Journal of Speech and Hearing Research* **6**, 111–128.

Sutton, N. G. (1971). "Anatomy of the Brain and Spinal Medulla" London: Butterworths.

Szent-Györgyi, A. (1953). "Chemical Physiology of Contraction in Body and Heart Muscle" New York, London: Academic Press.

Tarkhan, A. A. (1936). Ein experimenteller Beitrag zur Kenntnis der Proprioceptiven Innervation der Zunge, *Zeitschrift für Anatomie und Entwicklungsgeschichte* **105**, 349–358.

Tatham, M. A. A. (1969). The control of muscles in speech, "Occasional Papers" 3, pp. 23–41 (University of Essex, Language Centre).

Tatham, M. A. A. and Morton, K. (1972). Context-sensitivity in some electromyographic signals from *M. Orbicularis Oris*, "Occasional Papers" 12, pp. 32–49 (University of Essex, Language Centre).

Templin, M. C. (1957). "Certain Language Skills in Children: Their Development and Interrelationships" Minneapolis: University of Minnesota Press.

Van den Berg, J. (1958). Myoelastic-aerodynamic theory of voice production, *Journal of Speech and Hearing Research* **1**, 227–244.

Van den Berg, J. and Tan, T. S. (1959). Results of experiments with human larynxes, *Practica oto-rhino-laryngologica* **21**, 425–450.

Van Riper, C. and Irwin, J. V. (1958). "Voice and Articulation" New Jersey: Prentice-Hall.

Von Leden, H. and Moore, P. (1961). The mechanics of the cricoarytenoid joint, *Archives of Otolaryngology* **73**, 541–550.

Wade, O. L. (1954). Movements of the thoracic cage and diaphragm in respiration, *Journal of Physiology* **124**, 193–212.

Warren, D. W. and Du Bois, A. B. (1964). A pressure-flow technique for measuring velopharyngeal orifice area during continuous speech, *Cleft Palate Journal* **1**, 52–71.

Weddell, G. (1960). Studies related to the mechanism of common sensibility, *In* "Advances in Biology of Skin I: Cutaneous Innervation" (Ed. W. Montagna) pp. 112–159 London: Pergamon Press.

Weiss, C. E. (1969). The effects of disrupted linguapalatal taction on articulation, *Journal of Communication Disorders* **2**, 14–19.

Wever, E. G. (1949). "Theory of Hearing" New York: John Wiley and Sons.

Whitaker, H. (1969). "On the Representation of Language in the Human Brain" Working Papers in Phonetics, Department of Linguistics, UCLA, 12.

Wildman, A. J. (1961). Analysis of tongue, soft palate and pharyngeal wall movement, *American Journal of Orthodontics* **47**, 439–461.

Winkelmann, R. K. (1960). Similarities in cutaneous nerve end-organs, *In* "Advances in Biology of Skin, Vol. 1: Cutaneous Innervation" (Ed. W. Montagna) pp. 48–62 London: Pergamon Press.

Woodford, L. D. (1964). "Oral Stereognosis" MSc thesis in Orthodontics Chicago, University of Illinois at the Medical Centre.

Zemlin, W. R. (1968). "Speech and Hearing Science; Anatomy and Physiology" New Jersey: Prentice-Hall.

# Suggestions for Further Reading

For those students who wish to pursue further the subject matter in this book, the following list of publications may be useful. Those books listed under (A) are of a general anatomical and physiological nature, those under (B) are specifically concerned with the anatomy and physiology of the speech and hearing mechanisms.

## A

Bourne, G. H. (Ed.) (1972). "The Structure and Function of Muscle" 2nd edn Vols 1 and 2 London, New York: Academic Press.

Bowsher, D. (1970). "Introduction to the Anatomy and Physiology of the Nervous System 2nd edn Oxford: Blackwell Scientific Publications.

Cunningham, D. J. (1972). "Cunningham's Textbook of Anatomy" 11th edn (Ed. G. J. Romanes) London: Oxford University Press.

Davson, H. (1970). "A Textbook of General Physiology" 4th edn London: Churchill Livingstone.

Eccles, J. C. (1973). "The Understanding of the Brain" New York: McGraw-Hill Book Co. Ltd.

Feneis, H. (1974). "Anatomisches Bildwörterbuch", 4 verlag Stuttgart: Georg Thieme.

Passmore, R. and Robson, J. S. (Eds.) (1973). "Companion to Medical Studies" Vol. 1. Oxford: Blackwell Scientific Publications.

Keele, C. A. and Neil, E. (rev.) (1971). "Samson Wright's Applied Physiology" 12 edn London: Oxford University Press.

Roberts, T. D. M. (1966). "Basic Ideas in Neurophysiology" London: Butterworths.

Ruch, T. C. and Patton, H. D. (Eds) (1965). "Physiology and Biophysics" 19th edn Philadelphia and London: W. B. Saunders.

## B

Judson, L. S. V. and Weaver, A. T. (1965). "Voice science" 2nd edn New York: Appleton-Century-Crofts.

Kaplan, H. M. (1971). "Anatomy and Physiology of Speech" 2nd edn New York: McGraw-Hill Book Co. Ltd.

Minifie, F. D., Hixon, T. J. and Williams, F. (Eds) (1973). "Normal Aspects of Speech, Hearing and Language" New Jersey: Prentice-Hall.

Van Riper, C. and Irwin, J. V. (1958). "Voice and Articulation" New Jersey: Prentice-Hall.

Zemlin, W. R. (1968). "Speech and Hearing Science: Anatomy and Physiology" New Jersey: Prentice-Hall.

# THE INTERNATIONAL PHONETIC ALPHABET.

## (Revised to 1951.)

### CONSONANTS

| | Bi-labial | Labio-dental | Dental and Alveolar | Retroflex | Palato-alveolar | Alveolo-palatal | Palatal | Velar | Uvular | Pharyngal | Glottal |
|---|---|---|---|---|---|---|---|---|---|---|---|
| Plosive | p b | | t d | ʈ ɖ | | | c ɟ | k g | q ɢ | | ʔ |
| Nasal | m | ɱ | n | ɳ | | | ɲ | ŋ | N | | |
| Lateral Fricative | | | ɬ ɮ | | | | | | | | |
| Lateral Non-fricative | | | l | ɭ | | | ʎ | | | | |
| Rolled | | | r | | | | | | ʀ | | |
| Flapped | | | ɾ | ɽ | | | | | ʀ | | |
| Fricative | ɸ β | f v | θ ð s z ʃ ɹ | ʂ ʐ | ʃ ʒ | ɕ ʑ | ç j | x ɣ | χ ʁ | ħ ʕ | h ɦ |
| Frictionless Continuants and Semi-vowels | w ɥ | ʋ | ɹ | | | | j (ɥ) | (w) | ʁ | | |

### VOWELS

| | | Front | Central | Back | |
|---|---|---|---|---|---|
| Close | (y ʉ u) | i y | ɨ ʉ | ɯ u | |
| Half-close | (ø o) | e ø | ɘ | ɤ o | |
| Half-open | (œ ɔ) | ɛ œ | ɜ | ʌ ɔ | |
| Open | (ɒ) | a | æ | ɑ ɒ | |

(Secondary articulations are shown by symbols in brackets.)

OTHER SOUNDS.—Palatalized consonants: ʃ, ʒ, etc.; palatalized ʃ, ʒ : ɕ, ʑ.   Velarized or pharyngalized consonants: ɫ, đ, ẕ, etc.   Ejective consonants (with simultaneous glottal stop): p', t', etc.   Implosive voiced consonants: ɓ, ɗ, etc.   ɼ fricative trill.   σ, ʚ (labialized θ, ð, or s, z).   ƛ, ᵰ (labialized ʃ, ʒ).   ꜀, ʗ, ʘ (clicks, Zulu c, q, x).   ɺ (a sound between r and l).   ŋ Japanese syllabic nasal.   ƍ (combination of x and ʃ).   ʍ (voiceless w).   ɿ, ʮ, ɷ (lowered varieties of i, y, u).   ɜ (a variety of ə).   ɵ (a vowel between ø and o).

Affricates are normally represented by groups of two consonants (ts, tʃ, dʒ, etc.), but, when necessary, ligatures are used (ʦ, ʧ, ʤ, etc.), or the marks ‿ or ⁀ (t͡s or t͜s, etc.).   ‿ also denote synchronic articulation (m͡ŋ = simultaneous m and ŋ).   ɔ, ɿ may occasionally be used in place of tʃ, dʒ, and ʓ, ʑ for ts, dz.   Aspirated plosives: ph, th, etc.   r-coloured vowels: ɛɹ, aɹ, etc., or eɹ, aɹ, ɔɹ, etc., or ɛˠ, aˠ, ɔˠ, etc.; r-coloured ə : ɛɹ or əˠ or ɹ or ɚ.

LENGTH, STRESS, PITCH.— ː (full length).   ˑ (half length).   ˈ (stress, placed at beginning of the stressed syllable).   ˌ (secondary stress).   ˉ (high level pitch); ˍ (low level); ′ (high rising); ͵ (low rising); ˎ (high falling); ˏ (low falling); ˅ (rise-fall); ˄ (fall-rise).

MODIFIERS.— ˜ nasality.   ˳ breath (l˳ = breathed l).   ˬ voice (ŝ = z).   ˈ slight aspiration following p, t, etc.   ˔ labialization (n̫ = labialized n).   ̪ dental articulation (t̪ = dental t).   ˳ palatalization (z̦ = ʑ).   ˕ specially close vowel (e̝ = a very close e).   ˕ specially open vowel (e̞ = a rather open e).   ˔ tongue raised (e̝ or e̝ = ẹ).   + tongue advanced (u+ or u̟ = an advanced u, t̟ = t̟).   - or ˕ tongue retracted (i- or i̠ = i̵, t̠ = alveolar t).   ˔ tongue lowered (e̞ or e̞ = ẹ).   ˒ lips more rounded.   ˓ lips more spread.   Central vowels: ɪ̈(= ɨ), ü(= ʉ), ë(= ə̇), ö(= ɵ), ɛ̈, ɔ̈.   ˌ (e.g. n̩) syllabic consonant.   ˘ consonantal vowel.   ʃʳ variety of ʃ resembling s, etc.

# Subject Index